Occupational Performance Coaching

This book presents a definitive guide to understanding, applying, and teaching Occupational Performance Coaching (OPC). Grounded in principles of occupational therapy, person-centredness, and interprofessional frameworks of health and disability, this book will be of interest across health and rehabilitation professions.

Supporting people affected by disability to do well and live the life they want is the ultimate outcome of all rehabilitation professionals, no matter where on the lifespan our clients sit. Coaching is increasingly recognised as highly effective in achieving this aim. This accessible manual provides case examples related to diverse health conditions alongside practitioner reflections. Uniquely, this manual presents coaching methods designed specifically for the rehabilitation environment. This book is a manual for practitioners, researchers, students, and lecturers interested in gaining a robust understanding of OPC methods, theoretical basis, and implementation.

An e-Resource linked to this book provides access to video demonstrations, a podcast from Dr Graham, and downloadable materials including a self-assessment of OPC skills (OPC Fidelity Measure), templates for clinical work, and teaching presentation material.

Fiona Graham is Senior Lecturer in interprofessional rehabilitation at the University of Otago, New Zealand. Fiona has over 25 years' experience working with children and families in public, private, health, and education sectors. She travels internationally, speaking and teaching on the use of coaching in rehabilitation settings. Dr Graham developed Occupational Performance Coaching as part of her doctoral studies with Vale Professor Sylvia Rodger and Professor Jenny Ziviani at The University of Queensland. Her research continues to examine the use of OPC in diverse settings, knowledge translation, and interprofessional practice.

Ann Kennedy-Behr is Senior Lecturer in occupational therapy at the University of South Australia. An experienced clinician, she is passionate about supporting parents and caregivers of children with disabilities and making healthcare as accessible as possible, particularly for people living in rural and remote areas.

Jenny Ziviani is Professor of Occupational Therapy at The University of Queensland with extensive experience in family-centred multi-disciplinary research for children with developmental challenges and their families. Her specific interest is in strategies that harness motivation and support self-competence as children and their families navigate their way to achieving personally meaningful life goals.

Occupational Performance Coaching

A Manual for Practitioners and Researchers

FIONA GRAHAM,
ANN KENNEDY-BEHR
AND JENNY ZIVIANI

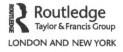

Routledge
Taylor & Francis Group

LONDON AND NEW YORK

First published 2021
by Routledge
2 Park Square, Milton Park, Abingdon, Oxon OX14 4RN

and by Routledge
52 Vanderbilt Avenue, New York, NY 10017

Routledge is an imprint of the Taylor & Francis Group, an informa business

© 2021 Fiona Graham, Ann Kennedy-Behr and Jenny Ziviani

British Library Cataloguing-in-Publication Data
A catalogue record for this book is available from the British Library

Library of Congress Cataloging-in-Publication Data
Names: Graham, Fiona (Senior lecturer in interprofessional rehabilitation),
    author. | Kennedy-Behr, Ann, 1971– author. | Ziviani, Jenny, author.
Title: Occupational performance coaching : a manual for practitioners and
    researchers / Fiona Graham, Ann Kennedy-Behr, Jenny Ziviani.
Description: Abingdon, Oxon ; New York, NY : Routledge, 2020. | Includes
    bibliographical references and index. | Summary: "This book presents a
    definitive guide to understanding, applying and teaching Occupational
    Performance Coaching (OPC). Grounded in principles of occupational
    therapy, person-centredness and interprofessional frameworks of health
    and disability, this book will be of interest across health and rehabilitation
    professions"—Provided by publisher.
Identifiers: LCCN 2020011504 (print) | LCCN 2020011505 (ebook) |
    ISBN 9780367427962 (paperback) | ISBN 9780367152253 (hardback) |
    ISBN 9780429055805 (ebook)
Subjects: LCSH: Occupational therapy—Handbooks, manuals, etc.
Classification: LCC RM735.3 .G73 2020 (print) | LCC RM735.3 (ebook) |
    DDC 615.8/515—dc23
LC record available at https://lccn.loc.gov/2020011504
LC ebook record available at https://lccn.loc.gov/2020011505

ISBN: 978-0-367-15225-3 (hbk)
ISBN: 978-0-367-42796-2 (pbk)
ISBN: 978-0-429-05580-5 (ebk)

Typeset in Vectora LH
by Apex CoVantage, LLC

Visit the eResource: www.routledge.com/9780367427962/eResource

In fond memory of Professor Sylvia Rodger: mentor, colleague, and friend.

Contents

Figures

Tables

Boxes

Foreword

I distinctly remember the 'Eureka effect' that I felt when I first read Dr Fiona
Graham's original article about Occupational Performance Coaching in 2010. At the
time, the literature was congested with ideas about how to change children and
how clinicians could be family-centred within therapeutic interactions. Whilst these
interventions and values are important, they squarely position clinicians as expert
advisors on healthcare solutions. As a clinical trialist, I have dedicated my career
to discovering what works best for children with disabilities and their families and
have sought to understand what helps children and parents to be the best versions
of themselves. What struck me about Graham, Rodger, and Ziviani's original case
reports was that they had scientifically validated the essential role of capacity
building for parents of children with disabilities – perhaps the most important
thing we ever do as clinicians. Their coaching research has moved the needle from
perceiving conversations with parents as 'non-billable cups of tea' to investing in
the person who knows and loves the child the best, galvanising parents' agency
to expedite their child's achievements. Over the years, I have had the privilege of
collaborating with, and learning from, these extraordinary authors, occupational
therapists, and women; whose humility, grace, and wisdom exemplifies the
greatest leadership in our field.

In any Olympic medal ceremony, winning athletes almost always thank their coach
first. Even though the athlete physically did the training and 'ran' the race, athletes
acknowledge the critical role that their coach plays in refining, strategising, and
motivating a win. No such accolades or recognition exists for parents of children
with a disability. Nor is there a coaching manual or an institute for intensive
learning. Instead, many parents tell me that the journey is isolating and stressful
and relies on persistently asking questions and anxiously striving to be the best
parent they can be. Yet all clinicians recognise that a parent's mental health,
capabilities, and belief systems have a profound effect on transforming a child's
outcome.

All of us will recollect a clinical scenario where we believed we could do more for the child, if only the health system would afford us more face-to-face therapy time. This book provides a refreshingly alternative clinical pathway, where the clinician's expertise shifts away from how they can personally help to fostering engagement with families that strengthens parental expertise and sense of agency. The Occupational Performance Coaching model is underpinned by three of my favoured mind-sets: compassion, curiosity, and learning. Therapists *connect* through high-trust partnerships founded upon mindful listening; then they *structure* and empower client-led goal setting and action taking to achieve goals; and finally, they *share* information in ways that amplify clients' awareness of their existing knowledge to foster personal insights. The artful conversation and compassionate, empathic partnership is designed to help parents develop a deep trust of themselves to solve their own challenges. Ultimately, this type of therapeutic exchange enables parents to solve problems independently without a reliance on clinical services, which may not always be available at the right time and intensity. Importantly, the model can be operationalised in multiple modes: face to face, over the phone, and via videoconference, making the intervention accessible to the most remote and vulnerable families. I am also excited that the known effective dose of four to twelve sessions is affordable and feasible to implement within our existing health systems.

This book is a must read for every clinician who ponders how they could do more to help. It challenges traditional views about our professional role. We are invited to experience the deep joy of witnessing the client-led goal achievement that comes from enacting an 'ask don't tell' mode of practice.

Iona Novak
Professor and Head of Research
Cerebral Palsy Alliance
Brain Mind Centre
The University of Sydney
Australia

Preface

We welcome the reader to this text explaining Occupational Performance Coaching (OPC) (Graham, Rodger, & Ziviani, 2009). This book has been prompted by the many practitioners, researchers, and students who have asked for an in-depth guide to the concepts, techniques, and application of OPC. Our exchanges with practitioners have also urged us to share resources which make implementing OPC easier in what are usually busy and complex work environments.

This book is intended as a guide to those new to OPC and those who may be familiar with OPC through training courses and published research. In this book we guide the learner to greater depths of understanding in the methods and application of OPC than have previously been available. Numerous new OPC resources are presented to aid understanding and implementation of OPC, including access to demonstration videos of Fiona with clients with a range of health conditions and cultural backgrounds and presentation materials for those introducing others to OPC (see eResources). Fiona also shares some of her personal journey to OPC in a podcast created for this book (see eResources).

This book represents a collaboration between Dr Fiona Graham, the original author of OPC, co-editors, co-authors, and contributing practitioners. Dr Ann Kennedy-Behr, as co-editor, was an early adopter and is a published author of OPC. Ann also authored Chapter 6 in which the research evidence for OPC is summarised. Professor Jenny Ziviani co-supervised Fiona Graham during her PhD studies and has co-authored several publications on OPC since that time. Chapters 2, 3, and 4 are co-authored by Fiona and Jenny. Sadly, Professor Sylvia Rodger, who also supervised Fiona's PhD, died in 2017. This book is dedicated to her. Dr Dorothy Kessler, a published author of OPC, co-authored Chapter 5 and informally contributed to discussions throughout the drafting of this book.

Graham, F., Rodger, S., & Ziviani, J. (2009). Coaching parents to enable children's participation: An approach for working with parents and their children. *Australian Occupational Therapy Journal, 56*(1), 16–23. doi:10.1111/j.1440-1630.2008.00736.x

Acknowledgements

This book has been made richer through the contribution of experienced practitioners and early adopters of OPC. These practitioners have openly and honestly shared their reflections on learning and applying OPC and provided feedback on the implementation resources provided within this book. A heartfelt thank you, therefore, to Charmaine Bernie, Lucy Charles, Arul Hamill, Penny Price, Kay Boon, Cheree Taylor, Shannon Pike, Chrisdell McLaren, Phoebe Griffin, Carmit Frisch, Caroline Hui, Aine O'Dea, Deirdre Fitzgerald, Cherie LeLievre, Dorothy Kessler, Melissa Nott, and Chi-Wen (Will) Chien.

Thank you also to Dr Chi-Wen (Will) Chien, Dr Mel Nott, and Dr Dorothy Kessler for their contribution to the development of the OPC Fidelity Measure (see Appendix A). Our ability to communicate many of the ideas presented in this book have been enriched through the skilful creation of graphics by Lance Nicholl, to whom we are very grateful.

A special thanks to Dr Laura Bergade (nee Desha) for her exceptional skills in project managing the preparation of this book; her ability to alternately adopt the lenses of student, practitioner, lecturer, and researcher were invaluable. This book would not be what it is without her.

Finally, this book would not have been possible without the patience of Fiona's children, Theo, Autumn, and Toby – thank you.

Abbreviations

ACT	Acceptance Commitment Therapy
ARC	Autonomy Relatedness Competence
ASD	Autism Spectrum Disorder
CC	Creative Commons
CEI	Coaching in Early Intervention
CI/OBC	Contextual Intervention/Occupation Based Coaching
CMOP-E	Canadian Model of Occupational Performance and Engagement
CO-OP	Cognitive Orientation to Daily Occupational Performance
COPCA	Coping and Caring for Infants with Special Needs
COPM	Canadian Occupational Performance Measure
CP	Cerebral Palsy
CPA	Collaborative Performance Analysis
DCD	Developmental Co-ordination Disorder
EBP	Evidence-based Practice
GAME	Goal Activity Motor Enrichment
GAS	Goal Attainment Scaling
ICF	International Classification of Functioning, Disability and Health
IDT	Inter-disciplinary Team
MBQ	Mealtime Behavior Questionnaire
MCHFS	Montreal Children's Hospital Feeding Scale
MDT	Multi-disciplinary Team
MI	Motivational Interviewing
MS	Multiple Sclerosis
OPC	Occupational Performance Coaching
OPC-FM	Occupational Performance Coaching Fidelity Measure
P4C	Partnering For Change
PEO	Person-Environment-Occupation Model
POET	Parental Occupational Executive Training
PREP	Pathways and Resources for Engagement and Participation

PRPP	Perceive Recall Plan Perform
RCT	Randomised Controlled Trial
RNLI	Reintegration to Normal Living Index
SDT	Self-Determination Theory
SFC-Paeds	Solution-focused Coaching Paeds
SMART	Specific Measurable Achievable Realistic Time-limited
TDT	Trans-disciplinary Team
TIDieR	Template for Intervention Description and Replication

Chapter 1
Introduction

Fiona Graham

Coaching has attracted considerable interest and attention as a strategy for working with clients in health and rehabilitation contexts in recent years, as evidenced by the high number of systematic reviews (Dejonghe, Becker, Froboese, & Schaller, 2017; Elek & Page, 2019; King & Xu, 2019; Ogourtsova, O'Donnell, De Souza Silva, & Majnemer, 2019; Tomeny, McWilliam, & Tomeny, 2019; Veen, Bovendeert, Backx, & Huisstede, 2017; Ward et al., 2019). Coaching has emerged as an effective element of interventions that achieve outcomes as diverse as employment for people with intellectual disability (Nevala et al., 2019), social and communication skills for children with autism spectrum disorder (Landa, 2018), and reduction in heart disease (Veen et al., 2017). Although the core elements of coaching are becoming well defined, this increase in popularity has also led to the ubiquitous use of the term coaching, in some cases confusing the distinction between coaching and usual care.

In this book we, Fiona, Ann, and Jenny, present one form of coaching, Occupational Performance Coaching (OPC), originally designed for use in rehabilitation settings by occupational therapists, with parents of children, who had goals for their children's greater engagement in occupational performance and participation in valued life roles. Today OPC is used across health and education professions with adults with a range of health conditions and/or caregivers of adults or children with health conditions. Throughout this evolution of the application of OPC, the outcome of interest has remained constant: client engagement in occupational performance and participation in life situations they value.

Occupational Performance Coaching is a goal-oriented approach in which client agency takes precedence in the selection of goals, analysis of situations, decisions about action to be taken, and evaluation of the success of those actions. In this regard, OPC is one of a wider family of coaching interventions in which the expertise of the health professional shifts from what they know about a client to their ability to engage with clients in a way that amplifies client expertise and agency (Baldwin et al., 2013; Kessler & Graham, 2015; Novak, 2014).

Occupational Performance Coaching is formulated as three hierarchically arranged and interacting domains of therapist actions: Connect, Structure, and Share (see Figure 1.1). First, drawing from the Connect domain, practitioner attention is on creating the conditions necessary for the formation of a high-trust partnership with clients. Mindful listening, non-judgemental acceptance, and authentic expression of empathy are consciously employed as part of this relationship development. Second, drawing from the Structure domain, the practitioner engages the client in a broad problem-solving process, orienting coaching conversations toward clients' personally valued goals. Client-led analysis of actions that could assist progress towards achievement of goals draws from any domain of life that the client perceives they could enact and that they think will work. This process starts by asking clients *"What is most important right now?"* Third, through the Share domain, the therapist draws on a range of strategies to amplify clients' awareness of their existing knowledge, to reflect on and thus gain insights into how things could be done differently.

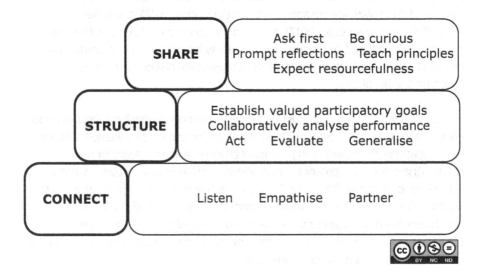

Figure 1.1 OPC three domains

Source: Figure 1.1 Three enabling domains of Occupational Performance Coaching. First published Graham, F. (2020), Occupational Performance Coaching Resources. Retrieved from www.otago.ac.nz/opc (29/01/2020). This work is licensed under a Creative Commons Attribution-NonCommercial-NoDerivatives 4.0 International License. University of Otago. Reprinted with permission.

Principles that underpin practitioner behaviours during OPC, and which are mirrored in the threshold concepts presented in Chapter 5, are:

1   High-trust partnerships are critical to effective help giving when the goals of working together are to participate more fully in life and society.
2   Clients are the agents of change in their own lives.
3   Meaningful goals are those that reflect clients' dreams – their aspired future states – rather than the minimisation of impairments or problems.
4   In the context of lifelong disability, sustainable goal-related change can arise from many systems and seldom arises from change to body structures and body functions.
5   Engaging with clients in ways that facilitate their sense of autonomy, competence, and relatedness is a distinctive and highly relevant skill in supporting achievement of occupational performance and participation goals.

In the context of a high-trust relationship and 'curious questioning' from the practitioner, clients' insight and creativity flourishes as they identify sensitive, novel, context-specific yet often very simple changes to the way they engage in goal-related activities. Change often starts with very small steps. Seldom do these changes require in-depth assessment of the limits of clients' abilities. Seldom does discovering these changes require a professional opinion of what the client can or can't do. Always, though, they require attention to what is meaningful, to what works, and a belief in clients' resourcefulness and competence. At times in clients' journeys toward achieving their goals, practitioners' health- and disability-related knowledge can be useful but far less often than practitioners may have assumed it to be, and only when permission to share is given by the client.

As a practitioner, attempting OPC can be fraught with uncertainty. *What kinds of goals might people come up with if I just ask them to name what is most important to them? What if their goal is not in my scope of practice? What if I do not think their goals are 'realistic'? If I ask clients what they think will work, they might get it wrong! They might think I'm asking because I don't know the answer, how embarrassing!*

Getting comfortable with this uncertainty has been a key part of the journey to becoming skilful at OPC for many of the contributors to this book, and none of us would say this is easy. Our professional enculturation as 'the expert' runs deep. Stepping into a professional situation in which we relinquish control over the agenda is no small thing to do. Our first attempts at OPC can feel like running towards a cliff edge strapped to a paraglider for the first time – totally nuts! Our feet, eyes, and sense of balance that have kept us upright on the ground all these years will be of almost no use. Yet we have a curiosity to do things differently, a sense that there is more to see than we have seen so far. Parachute affixed, we run to the edge of the field, the sky opening up before us as the land drops away. Our chute fills with air, changing all the sensations to our body – pulling us up rather than gravity weighing us down. It is terrifying. Then we remember the training. Pull here to go right and notice the subtle shift in direction. Watch the clouds, feel the wind. We realise that we are not without any control but that we can only respond to the elements and control this response – but not the outcome. We realise that we have resources – our training and our parachute, and that our sense of balance, our sight, and our legs are still useful, just used in different ways. Then we remember to look around. We can see from mountain to ocean; we look down on a flock of geese flying in formation. We see patterns we never knew were there – waves lining up to crash on the beach, crowds waxing and waning around an ice-cream stand with natural rhythm. All around is silence except for the wind. It is exhilarating. We are at the mercy of the wind and yet feel incredibly powerful. We know things now that we can never un-know. Landing is going to be a challenge. But we are getting the hang of this. It is feeling less strange. In an extract from an interview, Fiona describes her own experience of this journey into the unknown like this:

Fiona: When using OPC, I never know what's around the next corner; I'm not being the kind of guide who has already trod that mountain path a million times, and knows all the sites that are coming up . . . as if I knew exactly what [the clients] were going to see. With OPC, I don't know what they're going to see.

Interviewer: So you've let go of the control that you were talking about [earlier in the interview]?

Fi: That's been a huge part of my journey as a health professional, and a core attribute of somebody using OPC . . . an ability to let go of control. It's not that there is no control . . . OPC is not a sort of free for all . . . there's an element of guidance in there, but there's certainly a lot less control than what I see as 'usual care', even today.

Interviewer: That can be scary for a therapist.

Fiona: Oh, my goodness – incredibly scary! I remember one client, right at the time when I had started embracing what was really important to families, right now, as the starting point for therapy, and was [no longer] . . . cajoling their responses into some kind of nice answer that I was going to feel really comfortable with. This mum had a little boy, who had dyspraxia, learning disability . . . ADHD . . . and I just remember sitting there, I had the COPM [Canadian Occupational Performance Measure] open and was ready to write down the occupations that were most important to them, and then I just remember this da doof da doof da doof sort of sound. . . . It must have been my heartbeat or a pounding in my ears as the blood rushed to my head. I was just sitting there. Time seemed to stand still. And I just thought, "I have got no idea how to solve this problem. No idea what to do".

Interviewer: What *did* you do? What did you say?

Fiona: I sat with that feeling and it passed. It passed over. And then we started a conversation from there about . . . what we knew about how the child was going with the situation, and what we could do differently.

Interviewer: So it was a partnership?

Fiona: Partnership . . . exploring what some of the options were, and what was known already. What would work for her . . . what was known? And starting to work out what could work for this little boy.

You can hear more about Fiona's personal story of being confronted by this sense of uncertainty, ultimately arriving at OPC in a podcast (see eResources).

For those of us taking our first steps in truly client-led ways of working, OPC may be helpful – the equipment that allows us to fly. This book is your flight manual – a detailed guide to understand and implement OPC in varied health and education settings, from the perspectives of varied professionals. You may be a student of your profession, dipping in to OPC among many other interventions, looking for the 'feel' of OPC. You may have already had training in OPC or in other interventions that share some of the principles of OPC and several years' experience of working with clients. You may be a teacher of practitioners, or a researcher seeking specific information about OPC for specific purposes. We hope the organisation of the book makes this information easy to find. We hope that this book conveys the essence of OPC, prompts reflection on what you, the reader, currently know and how you currently engage with others when trying to assist them to move forward in their lives. Whatever knowledge, experience, and purpose the reader brings, we hope this book provides the necessary instruction in how to do OPC.

In Chapter 2, an overview of the theoretical and conceptual bases to OPC is provided, highlighting links between these theories and how each contributed to specific aspects of OPC. In Chapter 3, the three domains of OPC – Connect, Structure, and Share – are presented in detail with reflection questions and explanatory anecdotes provided throughout. Chapter 4 outlines the fidelity processes of OPC, explained in relation to undertaking independent research on OPC as well as clinical application of OPC in the way it was intended. The OPC Fidelity Measure

(OPC-FM) (Appendix A) is presented here and explained. In Chapter 5, readers are presented with five threshold concepts that are critical understandings to enacting OPC. Readers can access video demonstrations of each threshold concept by Fiona Graham and journey with practitioners' learning OPC through quotes shared by practitioners as they grasped each concept (see eResources). In Chapter 6, summaries of the research evidence on OPC to date, including its strengths, limitations, and questions yet to be answered, are presented. Then, in Chapter 7, this journey concludes with discussion of a range of issues that arise as OPC is implemented 'in the real world' of busy and complex practice environments. Practitioners with several years of experience implementing OPC share their lessons learnt, alongside our answers to frequently asked questions about implementing OPC – these are informed answers, but beyond what research can currently tell us. Presentation slides for non-commercial sharing of introductory information about OPC are provided along with other digital resources included in this book.

This book is designed to encourage different ways of engaging with material for readers with different learning needs and levels of familiarity with OPC. It is not anticipated that all readers will want to read the book from cover to cover, but chapters are arranged from background theory through to intervention details and research evidence, on to implementation experiences of practitioners. Within each chapter key messages are summarised and a series of reflective questions are provided to prompt the reader's deeper consideration of material and application of learning to their specific circumstances. A range of electronic resources, including video demonstration of OPC processes, are also available (see eResources). We expect that most readers will have particular learning purposes in mind and therefore may wish to dip into particular sections of interest.

REFERENCES

Baldwin, P., King, G., Evans, J., McDougall, S., Tucker, M., & Servais, M. (2013). Solution-focused coaching in pediatric rehabilitation: An integrated model for practice. *Physical & Occupational Therapy in Pediatrics*, *33*(4), 1–17. https://doi.org/10.3109/01942638.2013.784718

Dejonghe, L. A. L., Becker, J., Froboese, I., & Schaller, A. (2017). Long-term effectiveness of health coaching in rehabilitation and prevention: A systematic review. *Patient Education and Counseling*, *100*(9), 1643–1653. https://doi.org/10.1016/j.pec.2017.04.012

Elek, C., & Page, J. (2019). Critical features of effective coaching for early childhood educators: A review of empirical research literature. *Professional Development in Education*, *45*(4), 567–585. https://doi.org/10.1080/19415257.2018.1452781

Kessler, D., & Graham, F. (2015). The use of coaching in occupational therapy: An integrative review. *Australian Occupational Therapy Journal*, *62*(3), 160–176. https://doi.org/10.1111/1440-1630.12175

King, A., & Xu, Y. (2019). Caregiver coaching for language facilitation in early intervention for children with hearing loss. *Early Child Development and Care*. https://doi.org/10.1080/030 04430.2019.1658092

Landa, R. J. (2018). Efficacy of early interventions for infants and young children with, and at risk for, autism spectrum disorders. *International Review of Psychiatry*, *30*(1), 25–39. https://doi. org/10.1080/09540261.2018.1432574

Nevala, N., Pehkonen, I., Teittinen, A., Vesala, H. T., Pörtfors, P., & Anttila, H. (2019). The effectiveness of rehabilitation interventions on the employment and functioning of people with intellectual disabilities: A systematic review. *Journal of Occupational Rehabilitation*, *29*(4), 773–802. https://doi.org/10.1007/s10926-019-09837-2

Novak, I. (2014). Evidence to practice commentary. New evidence in coaching interventions. *Physical & Occupational Therapy in Pediatrics*, *34*(2), 132–137. https://doi.org/10.3109/019 42638.2014.903060

Ogourtsova, T., O'Donnell, M., De Souza Silva, W., & Majnemer, A. (2019). Health coaching for parents of children with developmental disabilities: A systematic review. *Developmental Medicine & Child Neurology*, *61*, 1259–1265. https://doi.org/10.1111/dmcn.14206

Tomeny, K. R., McWilliam, R. A., & Tomeny, T. S. (2019). Caregiver-implemented intervention for young children with autism spectrum disorder: A systematic review of coaching components. *Review Journal of Autism and Developmental Disorders*, *6*(3), 1–14. https://doi. org/10.1007/s40489-019-00186-7

Veen, E. V., Bovendeert, J. F. M., Backx, F. J. G., & Huisstede, B. M. A. (2017). E-coaching: New future for cardiac rehabilitation? A systematic review. *Patient Education and Counseling*, *100*(12), 2218–2230. https://doi.org/10.1016/j.pec.2017.04.017

Ward, R., Reynolds, J. E., Pieterse, B., Elliott, C., Boyd, R., & Miller, L. (2019). Utilisation of coaching practices in early interventions in children at risk of developmental disability/delay: A systematic review. *Disability and Rehabilitation*, 1–22. https://doi.org/10.1080/09638288.20 19.1581846

Chapter 2
Theoretical and conceptual foundations

Fiona Graham and Jenny Ziviani

Occupational Performance Coaching (OPC) is informed by several practice frameworks and theories of learning and motivation. These conceptual bases are reviewed in this chapter in order to clarify assumptions underpinning the application of OPC and mechanisms whereby change is proposed to occur (Hoffmann et al., 2014). We have chosen to present the theories that underpin OPC first; however, some understanding of OPC intervention components (described in detail in Chapter 3) may be necessary to fully understand the theoretical distinctions made in this chapter. Assumptions made throughout this chapter in relation to coaching are presented in a logic model at the end, linking theory, practices, intended client response, and outcomes. In recognition of readers' wide-ranging familiarity with the theories described later and possibly with OPC application, we encourage readers to move between sections of this book and not necessarily read from beginning to end. We hope that this chapter provides readers with an understanding of the core underlying principles and intended effects of OPC by positioning these within specific theoretical frameworks and models.

KEY MESSAGES

- Occupational performance and social participation are the outcomes of interest when applying OPC and are evident in goal statements. These outcomes have a critical organising effect on the application of OPC.
- OPC is informed by humanist principles of awareness and agency and a belief in the ability of people to make the best decisions for themselves. These principles influence several of the core therapeutic techniques within OPC as well as the mind-set of the practitioner when implementing intervention techniques.

- When working with parents of young children and caregivers of adult dependents, the family, and all its unique variations, is the unit of care in OPC. This means attending to the needs of the family unit and involving family members in working towards a goal, or working with family members separately.
- Addressing clients' psychological needs for choice and feeling cared for and believing in their ability to pursue their goals are core mechanisms thought to influence client engagement in OPC.

REFLECTIVE QUESTIONS

- Which theories currently influence the way you work? These may include profession-specific theories, or theories developed in relation to the client group or common health issue with which you work.
- If there were a common thread between these theories, what might that be? This link may be expressed as a philosophical statement, assumption, or intervention principle. It may be explicitly stated within these theories or be your own words and interpretation. Keep this in mind as you read through this chapter, and ask yourself how well each theory presented here aligns with the theoretical lens you already hold, and where each may bring something new. Consider if it would be helpful to integrate these ideas into how you view your work.

OCCUPATIONAL PERFORMANCE COACHING IN A NUTSHELL

Occupational Performance Coaching is an intervention for people with goals related to improving occupational performance and social participation in personally valued aspects of life. OPC is relevant for people and their caregivers, across the lifespan, who are experiencing restrictions in their ability to participate in life situations. This may apply to those with developmental, congenital, or acquired impairments to body structures and body functions, as well as environmental or personal restrictions.

Occupational Performance Coaching is largely undertaken as a coaching conversation between the practitioner and client/s with close attention to the development of high-trust relationships, in which the client is considered an active partner. The practitioner coaches the client through decision-making in relation to self-identified goals, analysis of performance of the goal situations, generation of ideas to move toward goal achievement, evaluation of progress, and generalisation of successful strategies. Practitioners' engagement with clients is guided by three domains – Connect, Structure, and Share – described later. Throughout the coaching process, emphasis is placed on the client's preferred future as the goal rather than the current problem situation, given the positive effect of doing so on identifying solutions. Strategies generated by clients are often novel as they emerge from clients' intimate understanding of their lives, abilities, environments, and value systems. The positioning of agency with clients (insofar as clients are able) is a priority within the therapeutic process. Clients deciding about what is addressed (the goal) and identifying and enacting changes in their lives are fundamental to clients' sustained investment in goal pursuit.

In this chapter, the World Health Organisation's framework for health and disability (the International Classification of Functioning, Disability and Health (ICF): World Health Organization, 2001) is first presented with particular attention to the concept of 'participation in life situations' and its relevance to goal setting in OPC. Second, the concept of occupation and occupational performance is discussed in relation to two models: the person-environment-occupation (PEO) model (Law et al., 1996) and the Canadian model of occupational performance and engagement (CMOP-E: Polatajko et al., 2007). The relationship between occupational performance and participation is then presented, with regard to the outcome of OPC. Third, person- and family-centred care philosophies are described alongside their influence on the way therapeutic relationships are constructed within OPC to support clients' autonomy, engagement, and sense of agency (Rogers, 1959; Rosenbaum, 1998). Coaching in OPC relies on a strong therapeutic relationship built on open communications, trust, and respect. Fourth, self-determination theory (Deci & Ryan, 1985) is explained as a basis for creating the conditions for sustaining client motivation even when the goals being pursued are challenging and complex. Only by developing confidence in one's ability to sustain goal pursuit can behaviours be practised by the client beyond the therapy contact time. Finally, adult learning theory is described as a framework for considering the role of clients as autonomous, self-determining learners, rather than their more traditional role as patients and recipients of care.

INTERNATIONAL CLASSIFICATION OF FUNCTIONING, DISABILITY AND HEALTH

The International Classification of Functioning, Disability and Health (World Health Organization, 2001) provides a means of conceptualising health, disability, and functioning (see Figure 2.1). The ICF has been widely adopted as a framework for

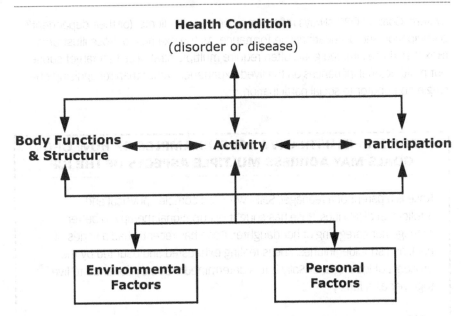

Figure 2.1 International Classification of Functioning, Disability and Health (World Health Organization, 2001)

interprofessional rehabilitation (Dean, Siegert, & Taylor, 2012; Stucki, 2005) and is presented here to explain some core concepts of OPC using inter-disciplinary language.

Within the ICF, a person's experience of participating in society is acknowledged as influenced by both biological and contextual factors, with neither alone accounting for an individual's successful and meaningful participation in society (Australian Institute of Health and Welfare, 2003). Within the ICF framework, *body structures and body functions* refer to biological factors, which represent function at the cellular level. The *activity* domain refers to a person's capacity to perform activities or tasks in ideal or controlled conditions, such as during therapy sessions. *Participation* considers the extent to which a person is able to participate in society (i.e., in societal or social roles) in ways and to the extent desired by that person. Participation is closely related to the concept of occupational performance within occupational therapy theory, with the two terms used interchangeably within OPC. *Contextual* factors which can influence a person's functioning are categorised as *environmental* (extrinsic to the person) and *personal* (intrinsic to the person).

Occupational Performance Coaching aligns with the ICF conceptualisation of health and disability as occurring in a complex (i.e., dynamic and interacting) system. Goals in OPC always reflect improvement in clients' (or their dependent's) participation and occupational performance. As the example of Rose illustrates (Box 2.1), these situated goals often require multiple strategies that target subtle but multifactorial influences on the lived experience rather than recognising one single contributor to social participation.

BOX 2.1   ILLUSTRATIVE CASE. EXAMPLES OF HOW OPC GOALS MAY ADDRESS MULTIPLE ASPECTS OF THE ICF

Rose is a parent of a teenager, Sally, who has complex physical and intellectual disabilities. Rose has sought occupational therapy to better manage her caregiving of her daughter. Rose has recently had a series of back and shoulder injuries. She is feeling exhausted and daunted by the prospect of looking after Sally but is determined that they continue to live together as a family.

Within a series of OPC sessions, Rose identifies her goal to 'maintain good health while caregiving for her daughter at home'. In progressing this goal, Rose might decide to improve her fitness or strength (*body structures/ functions*) if she identifies that this would improve her energy levels and minimise the risk of injuries to herself from lifting her daughter. She might also decide that accessing training in safe manual handling techniques (*activity/participation*) to improve her handling skills (*activity*) might help. Furthermore, she may consider asking her husband to share more of the caregiving role (*social environment*) or to access government funding for paid domestic assistance (*environment*). Her confidence in undertaking these changes is aided by her love of her daughter and her knowledge of her husband's love for his family (*personal factors*).

OPC targets participation outcomes

In OPC, the outcome of interest is always the client's occupational performance and participation in life situations (i.e., in valued daily life roles and tasks in the lived environment), hence, using the language of the ICF, goal statements in OPC always reflect a person's participation in life situations.

Within the ICF, *activities* and *participation* are intended to distinguish a person's *capacity* (i.e., ability to perform an *activity* under ideal or controlled conditions) from their experience of performing activities in the context of daily life (that is, their participation in society) (Australian Institute of Health and Welfare, 2003; World Health Organization, 2013). This is a critical distinction in OPC, as goals relate to participation rather than the execution of activities divorced from their real-world context.

Health and rehabilitation systems should focus on improving occupational performance and participation in the lived environment rather than on the more restricted intention of improving discrete, decontextualised task performance (Imms et al., 2017). Yet, several systematic reviews of rehabilitation research and clinical practice, with diverse health populations, indicate that even 20 years after the ICF was published, the majority of rehabilitation research and practice is still concerned with attempts to minimise a person's impairments or improve *activity capacity*, rather than their *participation* in valued social roles (Andringa et al., 2019; Ezekiel et al., 2019; Lee, Heffron, & Mirza, 2019). For populations experiencing ongoing disability or chronic health issues, there has been a shift in very recent years toward occupational performance and participation-focused interventions (Imms et al., 2016; Novak & Honan, 2019; Townsend & Polatakjo, 2013). OPC is now one of a family of such interventions that include coaching as a central therapeutic strategy to achieve these outcomes.

Several options for distinguishing between *activity* and *participation* intervention outcomes have been proposed (World Health Organization, 2013), and there is likely to be continued debate and clarification of this field (Imms et al., 2016). For the purposes of understanding the focus of OPC, the distinction between *activity* and *participation* is adopted whereby *activities* describe performance of tasks divorced from the lived environment (i.e., under ideal conditions and reflecting a person's *capacity*) while *participation* describes a person's participation in valued social roles and life situations in the lived environment (i.e., real-world conditions). In OPC, participation is conceptualised as the successful undertaking of core tasks essential to and illustrative of clients' successful participation in personally valued social roles. Improvement reflects the qualities of participation that clients value such as frequency, involvement, or satisfaction (Imms et al., 2016). Examples of these differences are provided in Table 2.1.

THE CONCEPT OF OCCUPATIONAL PERFORMANCE

While relevant to a range of health practitioners, OPC is informed by concepts and philosophies from occupational therapy. From an occupational therapy perspective, occupation refers to the context-specific activities of daily life that have inherent value and meaning to clients (Polatajko et al., 2013). Occupation is closely related to the concept of participation in the ICF as it shares a focus on involvement in

Table 2.1 Distinction between activity- and participation-focused goals

Activity-focused goals with no social context reflecting a person's capacity. (Not appropriate as OPC goals.)	Participation-focused goals embedded in the context of societal roles reflecting a person's performance. (Appropriate as OPC goals.)
John can tie his shoelaces.	John ties his shoelaces when getting ready for school at mum's house.
Jill can throw a ball.	Jill plays in the local netball team.
Mary can dress herself.	Mary dresses herself at home when getting ready to go out.

personally meaningful societal roles (Imms et al., 2016; World Health Organization, 2013). Occupational therapy is concerned with the use of occupation as a means (or mechanism) for regaining health and wellbeing and as the ultimate outcome of interest (Townsend et al., 2007). Occupational performance refers to the observed outcome of the interaction between a person, their occupation, and their environment (see PEO model in the next paragraph) (Law et al., 1996). Within OPC, occupation is reflected in the expression of goal statements as the performance of (and participation in) occupations (life situations). Clients are then coached through a collaborative analysis of performance of these goals, a process in which the activity focus, embedded in the contexts of life situations, is a central focus.

Occupational therapy has several models that describe the concept of occupation in the context of rehabilitation in health and social systems. Both the PEO and CMOP-E are appropriate models of occupation for examining and explaining OPC processes and outcomes. OPC was initially developed in line with one of the most conceptually simple models of occupation, the person-environment-occupation model (Law et al., 1996) (see Figure 2.2), in which the intersect of PEO represents occupational performance. The PEO depicts the relationship between a person, their occupations, and their environments and how these interact to influence a person's occupational performance. The environment includes influences close to a person such as the social and physical environment, as well as community-wide influences such as the cultural, political, and economic environment. The better the fit (or match) between a person's abilities, environmental demands and resources, and the complexity and valuing of the occupation, the greater (i.e., involvement, engagement, range, extent of) a person's occupational performance.

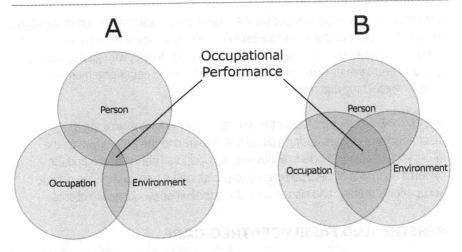

Figure 2.2 Person-environment-occupation (PEO) model

Source: Adapted from (Law et al., 1996).

In figure 2.2A this intersect is small, representing limited opportunity for the person to perform occupations successfully. In figure 2.2B, the greater intersect of PEO represents expanded occupational performance opportunity, affording a better match between the person, their occupations, and their environmental conditions.

A core premise of the PEO is that occupational performance improves when there is a good fit or match between the abilities and the support needs of a person, the demands of the occupation being attempted, and the extent of environmental supportiveness. This premise is applied within OPC with the notion of 'make it match', referring to prioritisation of achieving occupational success (i.e., enabling successful participation) as directly as possible (see Chapter 3). The PEO is often used with clients or in practitioner training in OPC to illustrate how change can occur in relation to client goals.

The Canadian model of occupational performance and engagement (Polatajko et al., 2013) is a more expansive theory of occupation that explicates the concept of engagement in the understanding of occupation. While consistent with the PEO, the CMOP-E expands on the three core concepts of person, environment, and occupation and emphasises the centrality of the client's value system (spirituality). Client engagement (investment, involvement, and immersion) in occupation is also highlighted to emphasise the relevance of the client *experience* of doing an occupation, rather than simply performing an occupation. This shift in emphasis on client experience as a key feature of occupational performance mirrors contemporary discussions about the ICF definition of participation, which highlights the need to consider the subjective experience of participation (Imms et al., 2017). Client values are central to the direction of coaching in OPC, with goals explicitly linked to client values with the intention of optimising client engagement in achieving coaching outcomes.

The CMOP-E provides a broader theoretical framework for examining the mechanisms of change arising from OPC compared to the PEO. However, the PEO can be a helpful model in explaining occupational performance and the systems approach of OPC, particularly to practitioners from disciplines outside of occupational therapy and also as a teaching tool when working with clients.

PERSON- AND FAMILY-CENTRED CARE

Both person- and family-centred care philosophies emphasise the importance of person (or family) uniqueness and involvement in health-related decision-making. Both philosophies are supported by large bodies of research evidence that link approaches drawing on these philosophies with high client engagement in therapy, satisfaction with therapy outcomes, and self-management of health (Dunst, Trivette, & Hamby, 2007; King & Chiarello, 2014; McMillan et al., 2013; Olsson, Jakobsson Ung, Swedberg, & Ekman, 2013; Rathert, Wyrwich, & Boren, 2013; Yun & Choi, 2019).

The use of the terms person- and family-centred care has become ubiquitous across health and rehabilitation services (Pryor, 2018). Have you met a clinician lately who has claimed to be unclient or unfamily-centred? Yet within resource-constrained systems, the application of these philosophies can seem opaque and reliant on a luxury of time that few health professionals feel they have (Turner-Stokes, 2007). Beyond the issue of time, clinicians describe a conundrum in which they must balance a desire to attend to participatory goals against medically dominant agendas of assessing impairments and attempting to 'fix' clients – in such a scenario, the client voice often loses its centrality.

Alignment of OPC with person- and family-centred care

The techniques and processes of OPC are consistent with person- and family-centred philosophy (King & Chiarello, 2014) and offer some ways to negotiate the diverse expectations of health systems. In OPC we work toward practitioner-client dynamics of practitioner as coach and client as active agent and self-manager. In doing so, the practitioner using OPC establishes a therapeutic context of creative, active problem-solving and self-monitoring of progress. In the next section, we describe person- and then family-centred care and indicate their influence on the development of techniques within OPC.

Person-centred care explained

At a time when psychoanalytic approaches dominated the field, Carl Rogers proposed what he called a patient-centred approach (now widely referred to as person-centred), in which the counsellor simply listened as people described their concerns, asked questions to encourage reflection, and responded to reflections without judgement. He termed this response 'unconditional positive regard' (Rogers, 1959). Clinician expression of empathy toward clients was also what Rogers considered key to effecting change with clients. Rogers observed clients' development of insight and adoption of new responses to longstanding problems when counsellors responded in these ways.

Person-centred care and its principles became widely adopted by rehabilitation professions as an alternative to 'illness-centred' care (Kogan, Wilber, & Mosqueda, 2016; Leplege et al., 2007). Occupational therapy integrated Rogerian philosophy in the early 1980s as a distinctive feature of the profession, widely adopting the term 'client-centred occupational therapy' as a professional by-line (Canadian Association of Occupational Therapists and Department of National Health and Welfare, 1983). Rogers's emphasis on recognising and valuing the 'whole' person was highly congruent with core occupational therapy views on the relationship between the whole (mind-body) person, their environment, and occupational performance (Law, Baptiste, & Mills, 1995).

Today a person-centred approach is widely considered the norm in many health professions (Brooks et al., 2019; Kogan et al., 2016; Yun & Choi, 2019) with descriptions of person-centred care emphasising partnership relationships, individualised care, and a bio-psycho-social view of a client and their circumstances (Santana et al., 2018). Outside of counselling psychology, person-centredness is often considered evident when shared decision-making between health professional and clients is observed (Dwamena et al., 2012).

Occupational Performance Coaching aligns closely with Rogers's original descriptions of person-centred care, in particular the relational elements, through the expression of empathy and non-judgement. When using OPC the clinician's initial objective is to establish a strong positive partnership in which the client feels valued, accepted, and understood. In OPC this partnership is coupled with a particular focus on clients' occupation and participation-focused goals.

Family-centred care explained

Several areas of rehabilitation, particularly paediatric rehabilitation (King, King, Rosenbaum, & Goffin, 1999; Visser-Meily et al., 2006), extended the concepts of person-centred care to the whole family. This extension of the unit of care recognises the centrality of family in childhood and during times of recovery from major illness during adulthood. Family-centred practice is universally considered best practice across children's healthcare and is considered an umbrella philosophy for all contemporary interventions related to children's development (Imms & Gibson, 2018). OPC is a family-centred intervention in that the subject of goals can be the whole family or any specific family member (such as parents, siblings, or child with a health condition) with an occupation and participation-oriented goal.

Culturally specific variations of person- and family-centred care also exist. For example, 'whanau-centred care' is often advocated when working with Māori, the indigenous people of New Zealand, whereby emphasis is placed on including the extended family (e.g., cousins, grandparents) within the unit of care. This approach reflects more culturally accurate definitions of family (Rochford, 2004). In principle, in OPC the unit of care is as wide as is meaningful to the client and over which the client has some influence. However, the extent of the unit of care (i.e., the individual, family/whanau or community) may be influenced by the service structure in which a clinician works, the nature of the health condition, or issues clients have. In applying OPC, it is critical that clinicians (and services planning service-wide use of OPC) are explicit about who the unit of care extends to, who it excludes, and that this is communicated clearly to all stakeholders.

*Coaching single and multiple clients: merging person-
and family-centred practices*

A key advantage of OPC as an intervention is that it can be applied at the individual or family level, thus it can be considered both person-centred and family-centred. The critical question of *Who is the client?* when more than one person is implicated in goals (such as both parent and child), is addressed in detail in Chapter 3 and in our earlier publications (Graham, Rodger, & Ziviani, 2015).

Building family capacity through coaching

In addition to meeting the needs of parents of children with disabilities, the notion of building family capacity (Chiarello, 2017; Dunst & Trivette, 2009) to self-manage situations has been emphasised as an important element of family- and person-centred care (Santana et al., 2018). Capacity building is reflected in the adage, "give a person a fish and they will eat for a day; teach them how to fish and they will eat for a lifetime" (Anon, https://knowyourphrase.com/give-a-man-a-fish). OPC is explicitly based on an intention to 'teach how to fish' with capacity building seen as a central long-term outcome. Capacity building goes beyond responding to clients' immediate needs to intentionally supporting the development of skills in self-management of their (or their dependent's) disability. Within OPC the emphasis on clients as autonomous decision-makers throughout all stages of OPC cultivates the skills and resources required for ongoing self-management thus building client capacity.

SELF-DETERMINATION THEORY

Client active involvement (i.e., engagement) in the therapeutic process is proposed as a central mechanism of OPC. Client engagement, in the context of OPC, includes clients' attention during therapeutic exchanges, their level of participation in decision-making, disclosure (honesty) with the practitioner, and willingness and ability to take action toward achieving their goals. If a client is unwilling or unable to engage with health professionals or to engage in the process of identifying solutions to their life challenges, then meaningful progress is going to be limited. Client engagement in any therapy is a transaction; that is, an exchange that involves the client, practitioner, and nature of the intervention. Client engagement is affected by clients' pre-existing psychological needs *and* how (and how well) the practitioner responds to these needs (Peter, 2019). In OPC we draw on self-determination theory (SDT: Deci & Ryan, 1985) to guide our understanding of client engagement and clients' ongoing motivation to pursue personally meaningful goals.

What is SDT?

Self-determination theory is a meta-theory of motivation (Ryan & Deci, 2017). From an SDT perspective, an individual's motivation to engage in an activity or behaviour is heavily influenced by the extent to which their psychological needs for *autonomy*, *relatedness*, and *competence* (ARC) are met.

The need to experience *autonomy* refers to a sense of personal agency, that we have an influence over our life course and situation. Perceiving that we have the opportunity and ability to make choices and to self-evaluate success or competence are important expressions of autonomy. The psychological need to experience *relatedness* refers to the need for connection with others, to feel cared for, and simply to share the sentient experience of being human with another. The psychological need to experience *competence* involves both having adequate skills to achieve a task and perceiving that one has the skills.

Practitioners using OPC strive to meet these psychological needs during every therapeutic encounter. The way we respond to clients has a significant effect on their engagement in therapy and motivation to make changes in their lives. OPC emphasises the use of techniques that respond to and address clients' basic psychological needs for ARC, thus heightening the conditions for ongoing goal pursuit. The application of ARC-informed therapeutic strategies of OPC is provided in Box 2.2.

BOX 2.2 ILLUSTRATIVE CASE. ATTENTION TO CLIENT AUTONOMY, RELATEDNESS, AND COMPETENCE DURING OPC

A mother of a child with autism may perceive that she does not have the skills to manage her child's 'meltdowns'. In this scenario, the mother's psychological need for a sense of *competence* is not being met. Providing this mother with a list of well-intended strategies known to reduce the occurrence of 'meltdowns' is likely to further compound her low sense of *competence* if she interprets this as further evidence of what she should have known or should be doing better.

During an OPC session a practitioner, instead of providing advice, would ask about and listen empathically to the mother's experience. The practitioner's non-judgemental acceptance of the mother's narrative and her emotional state (e.g., withdrawn, hostile, tearful) builds the mother's trust in the practitioner and begins to meet her need for *relatedness*.

Using OPC the practitioner would question the mother with curiosity about how she avoids, diffuses, and copes with the child's meltdowns. Questions could include *"How do you cope when he loses it? When have you noticed the meltdowns are more/less likely to occur? Given what you know about your son, what situations are guaranteed to trigger a meltdown? Tell me about what is going on when he is at his best? When have you noticed he is most relaxed?"* The questioning occurs with patience and persistence by the practitioner, guiding the mother to reflect on her situation from multiple angles. The practitioner avoids providing advice, and instead asks questions that promote reflection, reframing, and insight into the goal situation. The mother may not initially appreciate the strategies she describes, but her ownership of the strategies is important to her development of *autonomy* as she retains maximal control of strategy development.

The practitioner's questions also elicit evidence of the mother's pre-existing *competence* in managing the child's meltdowns and brings attention to this. Doing so challenges the mother's self-perception as 'incompetent' in dealing with the child's meltdowns, providing evidence of her ability, resilience, knowledge, and resourcefulness. In response, the mother is likely to become more animated and attentive and to volunteer further strategies she could use but hasn't yet tried. That is, the mother becomes more engaged in resolving the difficulty for which she sought help. She is also more likely to follow her own good advice and enact the strategy, doing so with much more conviction than she would have if advised on what to do.

The three enabling domains of OPC – Connect, Structure, and Share (all outlined in detail in Chapter 3) – represent therapeutic actions that meet the psychological needs of ARC, thereby supporting engagement in rehabilitation and change processes (see Figure 2.3). Although clients' psychological needs, as proposed in SDT, are relevant across all OPC elements, the need for *autonomy* is addressed most directly by the Structure domain of OPC; the need for *relatedness* is most directly aligned to the Connect domain, and the need for *competence* is most directly met within the Share domain. First, the OPC domain Connect attends to clients' need for *relatedness* through the use of mindful listening and expression of unconditional empathy for the client's experience. In doing so the practitioner conveys a level of non-demanding emotional involvement in the client's current experience. Second, the OPC domain Structure attends to the psychological need for *competence*. In OPC, Structure is provided by guiding the client to identify their primary goal (i.e., hoped for outcome, desire, aspiration) and outlining a stepwise process to move towards that goal. These steps are described in more detail within the elements of the Structure domain. Third, the OPC domain Share attends to the need for *autonomy* through the use of questioning to situate decision-making about reflection, learning, and insight with the client, rather than the practitioner.

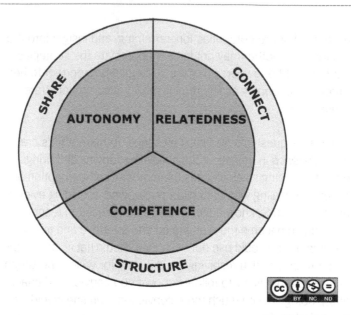

Figure 2.3 The relationship between the three basic psychological needs of self-determination theory: Autonomy, Relatedness, and Competence, and the three enabling domains of Occupational Performance Coaching: Connect, Structure, and Share

Source: Figure 1.1 Three enabling domains of Occupational Performance Coaching. First published Graham, F. (2020), Occupational Performance Coaching Resources. Retrieved from www.otago.ac.nz/opc (29/01/2020). This work is licensed under a Creative Commons Attribution-NonCommercial-NoDerivatives 4.0 International License. University of Otago. Reprinted with permission.

ADULT LEARNING

The aim of coaching is to support clients to learn new ways of interacting with the world in order to achieve personally valued goals. One useful way of thinking about coaching, then, is as a process of learning (Cox, 2015) and to think of clients as adult learners. Learning involves acquiring new information, relating it in some way to what is already known (so it is retained), then applying this information in some way; for example, adjusting future decisions or actions. Learning occurs during OPC, particularly as clients engage in a collaborative analysis of goal situations, reflecting on what influences their ability to realise goals, what their choices are in enacting changes, and how effective these changes are in relation to their identified goal/s.

Understanding and optimising the process of learning is therefore of interest when applying OPC. Thinking of OPC as a learning process, rather than a therapeutic one, can be helpful in shifting away from the historic power dynamics inherent in health professional-patient relationships. Ways of engaging with clients within OPC are guided by principles of adult learning as outlined by Knowles and colleagues (Knowles, Holton, & Swanson, 2005). In contrast to teaching and learning practices with children, Knowles and colleagues proposed that adult learners:

1   Need to perceive a reason to engage in learning and understand how learning is going to occur.
2   Need a self-directed approach to learning; for example, to have control over the pace and direction of learning.
3   Have life experiences that are varied, are numerous, and influence learning. Adult learners engage more deeply in learning when new learning relates to and builds on existing life experiences.
4   Integrate new learning when they are ready and recognise a need to learn.
5   Take a life-task specific approach to learning. Current life 'problems' are an important motivator for adult learners to engage in seeking and applying new information.
6   Are more motivated to learn by internal factors such as their values, perceptions, and enjoyment than through obedience to authority figures such as teachers or practitioners.

Overarching many of these adult learning principles are the concepts of autonomy and self-determination outlined earlier in the summary of self-determination theory. Adults (arguably, children as well) are more engaged in learning (and apply new learning) when they feel that the process of learning is overtly relevant to their current life experience and that they have a high degree of control over how learning occurs and is applied.

Alignment of OPC to adult learning theory

During OPC, the practitioner creates the conditions for learning (for example by asking questions that prompt reflection, reframing, and insight) and less frequently employs traditional didactic teaching methods, such as explaining. Any new information presented by the practitioner during OPC is directly related to clients' expressed desire for the information (their need to know and a current life-problem). For example, as a client describes her difficulty in assisting her wheelchair-dependent husband to get into the car, the practitioner might wonder if the client has tried using a transfer board. Rather than assuming that this will be the solution to the client's problem (or that the client will accept the solution), the practitioner using OPC would ask the woman if she was aware of some of the devices available to assist car transfers and if she was interested in trying any. While this exchange might seem time consuming, and in some cases might be unnecessary, inviting the client to choose (and potentially reject) new information is a powerful way of engaging an adult learner because it acknowledges their competence and authority over their learning needs.

Transformational learning theories

Transformative learning theory (Mezirow, 2000) is a specific adult learning theory which may have particular relevance to OPC. Transformative learning involves an emotionally supportive exploration of the evidence for beliefs and assumptions about a situation. Six themes common to transformative learning experiences are individual experience, critical reflection, dialogue, holistic orientation, context, and authentic relationships (Taylor, 2009). In relation to OPC, the themes of individual experience, holistic orientation, and authentic relationships are reflected in the OPC Connect domain, in which attention to and acceptance of the clients' experiences and perceptions is critical. The transformative learning theme of 'context' is consistent with the centrality of occupational performance and participation to OPC, centralising context in the expression of OPC goals. Critical reflection and dialogue reflect the processes within the OPC Structure domain.

The practitioner's role in facilitating transformative learning is to pay attention to the beliefs and assumptions conveyed in the client's narrative. Through a reflective discourse (Mezirow, 2000), the practitioner asks questions that invite the client to critically reflect on the evidence for their assumptions related to the expressed goal. This can be confronting and is sometimes emotional for clients (Taylor, 2009) given that new structures of meaning (i.e., core ways of making sense of the world) may occur. Within OPC the occupational focus of questioning on *what actually happens* allows this reflection to occur in a disarming, sensitive, but fact-focused way. The practitioner's emotional sensitivity, particularly the use of empathic and mindful listening, is essential to achieve the experience of emotional safety necessary for transformative learning to occur.

The profound (whole of life) change that is sometimes observed following OPC may be explained by transformative learning processes (Graham, Rodger, & Ziviani, 2014). During research on OPC, many parents of children with occupational performance issues were observed to reach a turning point at which it appeared that a core insight or shift in perspective occurred (i.e., a learning transformation) (Graham, 2010; Graham et al., 2014). Parents were often tearful just prior to, during, or after the turning point occurred. Parent dialogue prior to the session in which this turning point occurred were characterised by a focus on gathering information; 'problem-talk' (i.e., negative, hopeless, or blaming comments, seeking solutions from the practitioner); and isolated and superficial application of strategies. Conversely, the sessions following the turning point were characterised by parents reporting sudden improvement in children's performance of goal activities as well as improved behaviour and competence generally. For example, several parents commented that their children had 'just matured' subsequent to the turning point. When asked about the specific changes they had made to engender this change, parents were frequently more focused on reporting that they now *viewed* their children differently rather than describing what they had *done* differently. As parents came to view situations differently, it would be expected (from a transformative learning perspective) that their actions in all situations with children altered to fit the emergent perspective or new 'frame of reference' (Mezirow & Taylor, 2009). As occurred in the OPC study mentioned earlier (Graham et al., 2014), following the transformative learning process, a generalised change in performance, beyond the situations that were directly addressed, would be expected.

CONTRASTING OPC WITH OTHER COACHING INTERVENTIONS

The theories, frameworks, and models presented in this chapter as underpinning OPC collectively provide background to the arrangement, processes, mechanisms, and intended outcomes of OPC. Recent years have seen a wave of rehabilitation interventions with very similar foci on the way clients are engaged with and grounded in similar conceptual origins as described here for OPC. Rehabilitation is at an important transition point, in which attention to client engagement takes precedence over, or at least is equal to, a focus on impairments. Similarly, enablement of occupational performance and participation is more commonly a primary outcome, rather than an assumed consequence of interventions. Often, but not always, these interventions are called coaching or include coaching as a key aspect of the intervention, and many are summarised in recent reviews of coaching (Kessler & Graham, 2015; Ogourtsova, O'Donnell, De Souza Silva, & Majnemer, 2019; Schwellnus, King, & Thompson, 2015; Ward et al., 2019).

A brief summary of some of these interventions, highlighting key features, which enable comparison with and differentiation from OPC, is presented in Table 2.2. These interventions have not been selected systematically – the table is based on those interventions most frequently cited alongside OPC or raised with trainers during OPC workshops. The majority of comparison interventions to OPC are first proposed with paediatric populations, like OPC, and this is reflected in the interventions presented. For a more comprehensive list of coaching interventions related to rehabilitation, the reader is referred to

Table 2.2 Comparison of coaching interventions for children with developmental disabilities and their families

Intervention name (In order of year first published)	Population			Outcomes targeted				Assessment/Analysis			Intervention					Dose		Delivery	
	Infant/parent dyad	Child/Youth	Adult	Impairments	Normative skills	Occupational performance	Participation	Impairments	Environment	Activity/Participation	Envisioning	Client-led	Practitioner-led	Persuasive[1]	Direct education/instruction	Session Length (Mins)	# Sessions	In person	Tele-delivery
CO-OP[a]	-	✓	✓	-	-	✓	✓	-	-	✓	-	✓	-	-	-	50[2]	10	✓	-
CEI[b]	-	-	✓	-	-	-	✓	-	-	✓	-	✓	-	-	-	NS	NS	✓	-
OPC[c]	✓	✓	✓	-	-	✓	✓	-	-	✓	✓	✓	-	-	-	20–60	2–12	✓	✓
CI/OBC[d]	-	✓	✓	✓	✓	-	✓	✓	-	✓	-	✓	✓	✓	✓	NS	12	✓	✓
P4C[e]	-	-	✓	-	-	✓	✓[1]	-	-	✓	-	✓	-	✓	✓	–[3]	-	✓	-
SFC-Paeds[f]	-	✓	-	-	-	✓	✓	-	-	✓	✓	✓	-	-	-	NS	NS	✓	-
GAME[g]	✓	-	-	✓	✓	✓	✓	✓	-	✓	-	✓	✓	-	✓	30–90	18–30	✓	-
PREP[h]	-	✓	-	-	-	-	✓	-	-	✓	-	-	✓	-	-	NS	6–7[4]	✓	-
ParticipateCP[i]	-	✓	-	-	-	–[5]	-	-	-	✓	-	✓	✓	-	-	60	8	✓	-
BRIGHT[j]	-	-	✓	-	✓	-	✓	-	-	✓	-	✓	✓	✓	✓	45–60	14	✓	✓
COPCA[k]	✓	-	-	✓	NS	-	✓	✓	-	✓	-	✓	✓	✓	✓	NS	NS	✓	✓
POET[l]	-	✓	✓	✓	✓	✓	✓	✓	✓	NS	-	✓	✓	✓	✓	45	8	✓	-

Note: [a] Cognitive Orientation to Daily Occupational Performance (CO-OP: Polatajko et al., 2001). [b] Coaching in Early Intervention (CEI: Rush, Sheldon, & Hanft, 2003). [c] Occupational Performance Coaching (OPC: Graham, Rodger, & Ziviani, 2009). [d] Contextual Intervention (CI: Dunn, Cox, Foster, Mische-Lawson, & Tanquary, 2012) later called Occupation-Based Coaching (OBC: Little, Pope, Wallisch, & Dunn, 2018). [e] Partnering for Change (P4C: Missiuna et al., 2012). [f] Solution-focused coaching Paeds (SFC-Paeds: Baldwin et al., 2013). [g] Goal Activity Motor Enrichment (GAME: Morgan, Novak, Dale, Guzzetta, & Badawi, 2014). [h] Pathways and Resources for Engagement and Participation (PREP: Anaby, Mercerat, & Tremblay, 2017). [i] Participate Cerebral Palsy (CP: Reedman, Boyd, Elliott, & Sakzewski, 2017). [j] BRIGHT coaching (Majnemer et al., 2019). [k] COPing with and CAring for infants with special needs (COPCA: Akhbari Ziegler, Dirks, & Hadders-Algra, 2019). [l] Parental Occupational Executive Training (POET: Frisch, Tirosh, & Rosenblum, 2020). [1] Persuasive in this context refers to explicit attempts to encourage client agreement with practitioner's analysis or practitioner's strategy. [2] Dosage figures for CO-OP are based on 'classic CO-OP', however various dosages have been used with different populations. [3] As a tiered approach, P4C dosage is described as one day per week per school. [4] Session number is not provided for PREP but 6.5 hours of direct intervention per goal has been established (Dana Anaby, personal communication 23 December 2019). [5] The primary outcome of BRIGHT is family empowerment. NS Not specified.

Akhbari Ziegler, S., Dirks, T., & Hadders-Algra, M. (2019). Coaching in early physical therapy intervention: The COPCA program as an example of translation of theory into practice. *Disability and Rehabilitation, 41*(15), 1846–1854. doi:10.1080/09638288.2018. 1448468

Anaby, D., Mercerat, C., & Tremblay, S. (2017). Enhancing youth participation using the PREP intervention: Parents' perspectives. *International Journal of Environment Research and Public Health, 14*(9). doi:10.3390/ijerph14091005

Baldwin, P., King, G., Evans, J., McDougall, S., Tucker, M., & Servais, M. (2013). Solution-focused coaching in pediatric rehabilitation: An integrated model for practice. *Physical & Occupational Therapy in Pediatrics, 33*(4), 1–17. doi:10.3109/01942638.2013.784718

Dunn, W., Cox, J., Foster, L., Mische-Lawson, L., & Tanquary, J. (2012). Impact of a contextual intervention on child participation and parent competence among children with autism spectrum disorders: A pretest-posttest repeated-measures design. *American Journal of Occupational Therapy, 66*(5), 520–528. doi:10.5014/ ajot.2012.004119

Frisch, C., Tirosh, E., & Rosenblum, S. (2020). Parental Occupation Executive Training (POET): An efficient innovative intervention for young children with Attention Deficit Hyperactive Disorder. *Physical & Occupational Therapy in Pediatrics, 40*(1), 47–61. doi:10.1080/01942638.2019.1640336

Graham, F., Rodger, S., & Ziviani, J. (2009). Coaching parents to enable children's participation: An approach for working with parents and their children. *Australian Occupational Therapy Journal, 56*(1), 16–23. doi:10.1111/j.1440-1630.2008.00736.x

Little, L. M., Pope, E., Wallisch, A., & Dunn, W. (2018). Occupation-based coaching by means of telehealth for families of young children with autism spectrum disorder. *American Journal of Occupational Therapy, 72*(2), 1–7. doi:10.5014/ajot.2018.024786

Majnemer, A., O'Donnell, M., Ogourtsova, T., Kasaai, B., Ballantyne, M., Cohen, E., . . . Hanlon-Dearman, A. (2019). BRIGHT Coaching: A randomised controlled trial on the effectiveness of a developmental coach system to empower families of children with emerging developmental delay. *Frontiers in Pediatrics, 7*, 332. doi:https://doi.org/10.3389/fped.2019.00332

Missiuna, C., Pollock, N., Levac, D., Campbell, W., Sahagian-Whalen, S., Bennett, S., . . . Russell, D. (2012). Partnering for change: An innovative school-based occupational therapy service delivery model for children with developmental co-ordination disorder. *Canadian Journal of Occupational Therapy, 79*(1), 41–50. doi:10.2182/cjot.2012.79.1.6

Morgan, C., Novak, I., Dale, R. C., Guzzetta, A., & Badawi, N. (2014). GAME (Goals-Activity-Motor Enrichment): Protocol of a single blind randomised controlled trial of motor training, parent education and environmental enrichment for infants at high risk of cerebral palsy. *BMC Neurology, 14*(1), 203. doi:10.1186/s12883-014-0203-2

Polatajko, H., Mandich, A., Missiuna, C., Miller, L., Macnab, J., Malloy-Miller, T., & Kinsella, E. (2001). Cognitive Orientation to Daily Occupational Performance (CO-OP): Part III: The protocol in brief. *Physical & Occupational Therapy in Pediatrics, 20*(2/3), 107–123. doi:https://doi.org/10.1080/J006v20n02_07

Reedman, S. E., Boyd, R. N., Elliott, C., & Sakzewski, L. (2017). ParticiPAte CP: A protocol of a randomised waitlist controlled trial of a motivational and behaviour change therapy intervention to increase physical activity through meaningful participation in children with cerebral palsy. *BMJ Open, 7*(8), e015918. doi:10.1136/bmjopen-2017-015918

Rush, D., Sheldon, M., & Hanft, B. (2003). Coaching families and colleagues: A process for collaboration in natural settings. *Infants and Young Children, 16*(1), 33–47. doi:10.1097/00001163-200301000-00005

the systematic reviews of coaching referenced earlier. Further descriptions of OPC, linking theory, mechanisms, and outcomes and other features relevant to process evaluations, are also presented in the OPC logic model at the end of this chapter.

There are several similarities amongst the coaching approaches presented in Table 2.2 but also some important aspects of differentiation. An important step in further distinguishing amongst coaching interventions will be the development of fidelity measures for each. Fidelity measures will enable the capture of differences in the focus of practitioners' behaviours in each intervention, including items that highlight practitioner actions which are *not* considered part of an intervention (i.e., 'don't do' items). In the preparation of Table 2.2, fidelity measures could only be located for OPC, Pathways and Resources for Engagement and Participation (PREP: Anaby et al., 2017), Cognitive Orientation to Daily Occupational Performance (CO-OP: Polatajko et al., 2001), and BRIGHT coaching (Majnemer et al., 2019). The OPC Fidelity Measure is explained in Chapter 4 and provided in Appendix A.

The theoretical underpinnings of the interventions in Table 2.2 share similarities with OPC. All of the interventions emphasise clients in the contexts of their lives (e.g., grounded in ecological, dynamic systems and occupational theories), and all are described as either family- or person-centred. All interventions allude to the quality of relationships (e.g., client- or family-centred) but only a few – OPC, Solution-focused coaching Paeds (SFC-Paeds: Baldwin et al., 2013), and Participate Cerebral Palsy (CP: Reedman et al., 2017) – refer to theories that inform very detailed understandings of the transactive aspects of therapy (such as SDT: Deci & Ryan, 1985, described earlier) and provide guidance on interpersonal engagement with clients. All interventions echo OPC in encouraging autonomy-supportive strategies emphasising the centrality of client engagement. Of note, Solution-Focused Therapy (SFT) (also referred to as Brief Therapy) (de Shazer, 1984) and Motivational Interviewing (MI: Miller & Rollnick, 2002) have been cited as informing several of the interventions. Specifically, SFT elements are included in OPC, SFC-Paeds (Baldwin et al., 2013), and BRIGHT (Majnemer et al., 2019), while MI elements feature within Participate CP (Reedman et al., 2017). The link between SFT and OPC is described in Chapter 3. SFT and MI are not forms of coaching in themselves, hence are not included in the table; however, these approaches are briefly described here given their influence on the development of several coaching interventions emerging in rehabilitation.

SFT and MI have differing origins but are now applied with wide-ranging populations. Both are designed as brief (less than five) session interventions to support clients in adopting new behaviours. Both draw heavily on the use of empathy and development of strong therapeutic alliances, amplifying client autonomy and minimising the health professional-as-expert role. In SFT the clinician directs clients to envision preferred future states (and solutions whereby these can be achieved) rather than exploring current problem states. The 'miracle question' (described in relation to OPC in Chapter 3 of this manual) is a core technique of SFT and reflects a central focus on clarifying clients' goals (although the term 'goal' is avoided). Clients are encouraged to describe their strengths, resources, ways of coping, and exceptions to the problem in order to amplify their sense of competence to act. Effectiveness of SFT appears to be greater for mild or early stage psychological difficulty (Bond, Woods, Humphrey, Symes, & Green, 2013).

Motivational Interviewing is structured around four principles: express empathy, develop discrepancy (e.g., between client's current behaviour and their desired outcome), roll with resistance, and support self-efficacy. Distinctively, MI techniques amplify an internal ambivalence with current (unhealthy) behaviours and evoke client talk to amplify action toward preferred (healthy) behaviours through the sequence of questioning about positive versus negative behaviours. In contrast, SFT (and OPC) do not include strategies intended to influence the direction of client's decision-making.

All interventions include participation in life situations and/or occupational performance as a central outcome, along with reference to capacity-building outcomes (e.g., generalisation of learning, self-management) with the Canadian Occupational Performance Measure (COPM) (Law et al., 2005) most commonly used as the primary outcome measure for both occupational performance and participation outcomes. Occupational performance is the primary outcome of OPC, Goal Activity Motor Enrichment (GAME: Morgan et al., 2014), Contextual Intervention (CI: Dunn et al., 2012, later called Occupation-Based Coaching, OBC: Little et al., 2018), CO-OP (Polatajko et al., 2001), and Parental Occupational Executive Training (POET: Frisch et al., 2020). Only one intervention (BRIGHT coaching) is not described as addressing participation. Goal Attainment Scaling (GAS: Kiresuk & Sherman, 1968) is also often used in tandem with the COPM.

All interventions include goal setting and all but one include *activity/participation* analysis (POET: Frisch et al., 2020). All refer to processes as 'collaborative'; however, there are differences in the degree to which collaboration appears to be practitioner-led versus client-led. For example, interventions that commence analysis with formal assessments of clients' (or their children's/dependents') impairments (e.g., CI/OBC: Dunn et al., 2012; Little et al., 2018) and POET (e.g., PREP: Anaby et al., 2017) reflect a weighting towards practitioner-led analysis given that these require practitioner interpretation. OPC and SFC-Paeds (Baldwin et al., 2013) are distinctive in describing performance analysis as specifically client-led (supported by an absence of practitioner-led assessment) in response to reflective questions posed by the practitioner.

Distinguishing aspects of OPC from other coaching interventions

Occupational Performance Coaching is distinct in its application with dyads, adults, and youth, detailed instruction on relational aspects of coaching (i.e., the Connect domain), and explicitly client-led performance analysis (collaborative performance analysis), with detailed instruction on guiding clients in performance analysis. Despite all interventions being described as 'collaborative', some interventions, including COPing with and CAring for infants with special needs (COPCA: Akhbari Ziegler et al., 2019), POET (Frisch et al., 2020), and CI/OBC (Dunn et al., 2012), explicitly describe the use of directive strategies, applied with the intention of influencing client strategy development such as hinting, instructing, or lecturing on best viewpoint, interpretation, or actions. In the wider literature these kinds of therapeutic strategies are referred to as persuasive (Miller & Rollnick, 2012) or 'coercive' (Hall, Staiger, Simpson, Best, & Lubman, 2016), even when applied subtly. Given their distinct departure from alliance with the client and non-judgement, two central features of OPC, these strategies are noteworthy in a comparison of coaching-related rehabilitation interventions. The use of persuasion is explicitly listed as distinguishing (don't do) behaviours on the OPC Fidelity Measure (see Appendix A). While represented in the table categorically, the situating of authority (i.e., as expert and director of therapy) in these interventions is more accurately on a continuum between practitioner-led to client-led, with all interventions being more client-led than historic descriptions of rehabilitation interventions.

While all interventions allude to a relational focus – that is, specific attention to the development of collaborative relationships within the intervention, this appears to be more central to some interventions (including OPC, SFC-Paeds (Baldwin et al., 2013)) than others (e.g., PREP (Anaby et al., 2017), COPCA (Akhbari Ziegler et al., 2019)) given the degree of detail provided as to how relationships are fostered. Of those with greater emphasis on relational elements, most also refer to SFC or MI as component interventions (these including OPC, SFC-Paeds (Baldwin et al., 2013), and Participate CP (Reedman et al., 2017)).

The conceptualisation of client learning and intervention methods that support learning is one of the most diverse aspects of these coaching interventions. Learning is referred to in all interventions but with differences in emphasis on child learning, motor-learning, and adult learning. OPC and CI/OBC (Dunn et al., 2012) refer specifically to transformative learning within the family of adult learning theories. BRIGHT coaching was alone in including asynchronous online learning, with a pre-determined curriculum.

OCCUPATIONAL PERFORMANCE COACHING LOGIC MODEL

A logic model graphically illustrates an intervention including what is delivered, how it will be delivered, and the mechanisms through which an intervention is intended to affect outcomes, including possible mediators (Moore et al., 2015). A logic model is helpful when planning and reporting evaluation of an intervention by describing the features of an intervention clearly, including the

Table 2.3 Logic model for Occupational Performance Coaching

Arguments for OPC	Implementation criteria	Mechanisms and impact		Outcomes
		Practitioner resource (i.e., action)	Intended client response	
Occupational performance and participation are priority outcomes for many people living with disability and their caregivers. Usual care in rehabilitation has remained highly practitioner (expert)-directed despite evidence that client autonomy during rehabilitation results in higher client engagement. Interventions are needed that directly target occupational performance and participation as a primary outcome. Achievement of occupational performance and participation outcomes is multifactorial, requiring accommodation of individual and contextual influences.	In-person or web-based staff training in OPC www.otago.ac.nz/opc/training Self-audit through use of the OPC-FM or OPC Casenote Audit Tool. Delivered 1:1 or in groups; in person or via telehealth. Average dosage: 5 sessions (min 1: max 12).	PARTNERSHIP Explicit development of high-trust partnership. GOALS Identifying clients' most valued goal/s expressed as occupational performance and participation in life situations. AUTONOMY SUPPORT Client reflection, analysis, and decision-making encouraged. Client agency is maintained as paramount. SUPPORTING CHANGE Clients' specific action statements elicited.	PARTNERSHIP Client trusts practitioner thus reflects and discloses key information. GOALS A. Client undertakes independent goal striving. B. Detailed situation analysis by client. AUTONOMY SUPPORT Client experiences heightened autonomy over their goal situation thereby supporting intention to act. SUPPORTING CHANGE Barriers to action proactively addressed.	PRIMARY OUTCOME Individualised client goal achievement of greater occupational performance and social participation (e.g., as measured by the COPM or GAS). SECONDARY OUTCOMES High sense of competence, confidence, self-esteem, and self-management related to health condition/role/goal. LONG-TERM OUTCOMES Client and family capacity building and self-management.

proposed links between these. The model provides a summary of intervention components, thereby enabling researchers to examine data retrospectively to better interpret positive or negative findings. It also provides clarity as to how and under what conditions OPC intervention can be modified (i.e., tailored) when applied in different contexts, providing guidance to researchers intending to do this.

The OPC logic model presented in this chapter (See Table 2.3) specifies:

- The issues OPC is intended to address and arguments for OPC as a solution to these issues.
- The ways in which implementation criteria are identified for OPC, including the OPC Fidelity Measure, format of delivery, and dosage guidelines.
- The mechanisms and impact of OPC, including practitioner resources (otherwise known as the 'key ingredients') and intended client response.
- The intended short- and long-term outcomes of OPC.

CONCLUSION

This chapter outlined the major theories, models, and frameworks which underpin OPC and inform the hypothesised mechanisms that affect outcomes. Respect for and elevation of client sense of autonomy over the direction of therapy is a core theme linking each body of knowledge to OPC techniques and processes. Conceptualising client issues in OPC as activities performed or participated in within specific life contexts is also explained in relation to interprofessional and occupational therapy-specific frameworks, which acknowledge client success as influenced by dynamic and interacting systems. In the following chapter, the structure and techniques of OPC' to avoid confusion in use of the word 'structure' here, as not referring to the Structure domain.

REFERENCES

Akhbari Ziegler, S., Dirks, T., & Hadders-Algra, M. (2019). Coaching in early physical therapy intervention: The COPCA program as an example of translation of theory into practice. *Disability and Rehabilitation*, 41(15), 1846–1854. https://doi.org/10.1080/09638288.2018.1448468

Anaby, D., Mercerat, C., & Tremblay, S. (2017). Enhancing youth participation using the PREP intervention: Parents' perspectives. *International Journal of Environmental Research and Public Health*, 14(9). https://doi.org/10.3390/ijerph14091005

Andringa, A., van de Port, I., van Wegen, E., Ket, J., Meskers, C., & Kwakkel, G. (2019). Effectiveness of botulinum toxin treatment for upper limb spasticity poststroke over different ICF domains: A systematic review and meta-analysis. *Archives of Physical Medicine and Rehabilitation, 100*(9), 1703–1725. https://doi.org/10.1016/j.apmr.2019.01.016

Australian Institute of Health and Welfare (AIHW). (2003). *ICF Australian user guide.* Version 1.0. Disability Series. AIHW Cat. No. DIS 33. Canberra: AIHW.

Baldwin, P., King, G., Evans, J., McDougall, S., Tucker, M., & Servais, M. (2013). Solution-focused coaching in pediatric rehabilitation: An integrated model for practice. *Physical & Occupational Therapy in Pediatrics, 33*(4), 1–17. https://doi.org/10.3109/01942638.2013.784718

Bond, C., Woods, K., Humphrey, N., Symes, W., & Green, L. (2013). Practitioner review: The effectiveness of solution focused brief therapy with children and families: A systematic and critical evaluation of the literature from 1990–2010. *Journal of Child Psychology and Psychiatry and Allied Disciplines, 54*(7), 707–723. https://doi.org/10.1111/jcpp.12058

Brooks, A. J., Koithan, M. S., Lopez, A. M., Klatt, M., Lee, J. K., Goldblatt, E., . . . Lebensohn, P. (2019). Incorporating integrative healthcare into interprofessional education: What do primary care training programs need? *Journal of Interprofessional Education and Practice, 14*, 6–12. https://doi.org/10.1016/j.xjep.2018.10.006

Canadian Association of Occupational Therapists and Department of National Health and Welfare. (1983). *Guidelines for client-centred practice of occupational therapy (H39-33/1983E).* Ottawa, ON: Department of National Health and Welfare.

Chiarello, L. A. (2017). Excellence in promoting participation: Striving for the 10 Cs-Client-Centered Care, Consideration of Complexity, Collaboration, Coaching, Capacity Building, Contextualization, Creativity, Community, Curricular Changes, and Curiosity. *Pediatric Physical Therapy, 29*(Suppl. 3), S16–S22. https://doi.org/10.1097/PEP.0000000000000382

Cox, E. (2015). Coaching and adult learning: Theory and practice. *New Directions for Adult and Continuing Education, 2015*(148), 27–38. https://doi.org/10.1002/ace.20149

Dean, S., Siegert, R., & Taylor, W. (Eds.). (2012). *Interprofessional rehabilitation.* Chichester: Wiley.

Deci, E. L., & Ryan, R. M. (1985). *Intrinsic motivation and self determination in human behavior.* New York: Plenum.

de Shazer, S. (1984). *Keys to solutions in brief therapy.* New York: Norton.

Dunn, W., Cox, J., Foster, L., Mische-Lawson, L., & Tanquary, J. (2012). Impact of a contextual intervention on child participation and parent competence among children with autism spectrum disorders: A pretest-posttest repeated-measures design. *American Journal of Occupational Therapy, 66*(5), 520–528. https://doi.org/10.5014/ajot.2012.004119

Dunst, C. J., & Trivette, C. M. (2009). Capacity-building family-systems intervention practices. *Journal of Family Social Work, 12*(2), 119–143. https://doi.org/10.1080/10522150802713322

Dunst, C. J., Trivette, C. M., & Hamby, D. W. (2007). Meta-analysis of family-centered helpgiving practices research. *Mental Retardation and Developmental Disabilities Research Reviews, 13*(4), 370–378. https://doi.org/10.1002/mrdd.20176

Dwamena, F., Holmes-Rovner, M., Gaulden, C. M., Jorgenson, S., Sadigh, G., Sikorskii, A., . . . Olomu, A. (2012). Interventions for providers to promote a patient-centred approach in clinical consultations. *Cochrane Database of Systematic Reviews, 12.* https://doi.org/10.1002/14651858.CD003267.pub2

Ezekiel, L., Collett, J., Mayo, N. E., Pang, L., Field, L., & Dawes, H. (2019). Factors associated with participation in life situations for adults with stroke: A systematic review. *Archives of Physical Medicine and Rehabilitation, 100*(5), 945–955. https://doi.org/10.1016/j.apmr.2018.06.017

Frisch, C., Tirosh, E., & Rosenblum, S. (2020). Parental Occupation Executive Training (POET): An efficient innovative intervention for young children with Attention Deficit Hyperactive Disorder. *Physical & Occupational Therapy in Pediatrics, 40*(1), 47–61. https://doi.org/10.1080/01942638.2019.1640336

Graham, F. (2010). *Occupational Performance Coaching: An approach to enabling performance with children and parents*. Doctoral dissertation, University of Queensland, Brisbane. Retrieved from http://espace.library.uq.edu.au/view/UQ:229057

Graham, F., Rodger, S., & Ziviani, J. (2009). Coaching parents to enable children's participation: An approach for working with parents and their children. *Australian Occupational Therapy Journal, 56*(1), 16–23. https://doi.org/10.1111/j.1440-1630.2008.00736.x

Graham, F., Rodger, S., & Ziviani, J. (2014). Mothers' experiences of engaging in Occupational Performance Coaching. *British Journal of Occupational Therapy, 77*(4), 189–197. https://doi.org/10.4276/030802214x13968769798791

Graham, F., Rodger, S., & Ziviani, J. (2015). Coaching caregivers to enable children's participation: Whose goals are they anyway? In J. Ziviani, A. A. Poulsen, & M. Cuskelly (Eds.), *Goal setting and motivation in therapy: Engaging children and parents* (pp. 100–112). London: Jessica Kingsley.

Hall, K., Staiger, P. K., Simpson, A., Best, D., & Lubman, D. I. (2016). After 30 years of dissemination, have we achieved sustained practice change in motivational interviewing? *Addiction, 111*(7), 1144–1150. https://doi.org/10.1111/add.13014

Hoffmann, T. C., Glasziou, P. P., Boutron, I., Milne, R., Perera, R., Moher, D., . . . Johnston, M. (2014). Better reporting of interventions: Template for Intervention Description and Replication (TIDieR) checklist and guide. *British Medical Journal, 348*, 1–12. https://doi.org/10.1136/bmj.g1687

Imms, C., Adair, B., Keen, D., Ullenhag, A., Rosenbaum, P., & Granlund, M. (2016). "Participation": A systematic review of language, definitions, and constructs used in intervention research with children with disabilities. *Developmental Medicine & Child Neurology, 58*(1), 29–38. https://doi.org/10.1111/dmcn.12932

Imms, C., & Gibson, N. (2018). An overview of evidence-based occupational and physiotherapy for children with cerebral palsy. In C. P. Panteliadis (Ed.), *Cerebral palsy: A multidisciplinary approach* (pp. 165–192). Cham: Springer International Publishing.

Imms, C., Granlund, M., Wilson, P., Steenbergen, B., Rosenbaum, P., & Gordon, A. (2017). Participation, both a means and an end: A conceptual analysis of processes and outcomes in childhood disability. *Developmental Medicine & Child Neurology, 59*(1), 16–25. https://doi.org/10.1111/dmcn.13237

Kessler, D., & Graham, F. (2015). The use of coaching in occupational therapy: An integrative review. *Australian Occupational Therapy Journal, 62*(3), 160–176. https://doi.org/10.1111/1440-1630.12175

King, G., & Chiarello, L. (2014). Family-centered care for children with cerebral palsy: Conceptual and practical considerations to advance care and practice. *Journal of Child Neurology, 29*(8), 1046–1054. https://doi.org/10.1177/0883073814533009

King, G., King, S., Rosenbaum, P., & Goffin, R. (1999). Family-centered caregiving and well-being of parents of children with disabilities: Linking process with outcome. *Journal of Pediatric Psychology, 24*(1), 41–53. https://doi.org/10.1093/jpepsy/24.1.41

Kiresuk, T. J., & Sherman, R. E. (1968). Goal attainment scaling: A general method for evaluating comprehensive community mental health programs. *Community Mental Health Journal, 4*(6), 443–453. https://doi.org/10.1007/BF01530764

Knowles, M., Holton, E., & Swanson, R. (2005). *The adult learner: The definitive classic in adult education and human resource development* (6th ed.). Amsterdam: Elsevier Butterworth Heinemann.

Kogan, A. C., Wilber, K., & Mosqueda, L. (2016). Person-centered care for older adults with chronic conditions and functional impairment: A systematic literature review. *Journal of the American Geriatrics Society, 64*(1), e1–e7.

Law, M., Baptiste, S., Carswell, A., McColl, A., Polatajko, H., & Pollock, N. (2005). *COPM: Canadian occupational performance measure* (4th ed.). Ottawa, ON: CAOT Publications ACE.

Law, M., Baptiste, S., & Mills, J. (1995). Client-centred practice: What does it mean and does it make a difference? *Canadian Journal of Occupational Therapy, 62*(5), 250–257. https://doi.org/10.1177/000841749506200504

Law, M., Cooper, B., Strong, B., Stewart, D., Rigby, P., & Letts, L. (1996). The Person-Environment Occupation model: A transactive approach to occupational performance. *Canadian Journal of Occupational Therapy, 63*(1), 9–23. https://doi.org/10.1177/000841749606300103

Lee, D., Heffron, J. L., & Mirza, M. (2019). Content and effectiveness of interventions focusing on community participation poststroke: A systematic review. *Archives of Physical Medicine and Rehabilitation, 100*(11), 2179–2192. https://doi.org/10.1016/j.apmr.2019.06.008

Leplege, A., Gzil, F., Cammelli, M., Lefeve, C., Pachoud, B., & Ville, I. (2007). Person-centredness: Conceptual and historical perspectives. *Disability and Rehabilitation, 29*(20–21), 1555–1565. https://doi.org/10.1080/09638280701618661

Little, L. M., Pope, E., Wallisch, A., & Dunn, W. (2018). Occupation-based coaching by means of telehealth for families of young children with autism spectrum disorder. *American Journal of Occupational Therapy, 72*(2), 1–7. https://doi.org/10.5014/ajot.2018.024786

Majnemer, A., O'Donnell, M., Ogourtsova, T., Kasaai, B., Ballantyne, M., Cohen, E., . . . Hanlon-Dearman, A. (2019). BRIGHT coaching: A randomised controlled trial on the effectiveness of a developmental coach system to empower families of children with emerging developmental delay. *Frontiers in Pediatrics, 7*, 332. https://doi.org/10.3389/fped.2019.00332

McMillan, S. S., Kendall, E., Sav, A., King, M. A., Whitty, J. A., Kelly, F., & Wheeler, A. J. (2013). Patient-centered approaches to health care: A systematic review of randomized controlled trials. *Medical Care Research and Review, 70*(6), 567–596. https://doi.org/10.1177/1077558713496318

Mezirow, J. (2000). *Learning as transformation: Critical perspectives on a theory in progress*. San Fancisco, CA: Jossey-Bass.

Mezirow, J., & Taylor, E. (Eds.). (2009). *Transformative learning in practice. Insights from community, workplace and higher education*. San Francisco, CA: Jossey-Bass.

Miller, W., & Rollnick, S. (2002). *Motivational interviewing: Preparing people for change* (2nd ed.). New York: Guilford Press.

Miller, W., & Rollnick, S. (2012). *Motivational interviewing: Helping people change* (3rd ed.). New York: Guilford Press.

Missiuna, C., Pollock, N., Levac, D., Campbell, W., Sahagian-Whalen, S., Bennett, S., . . . Russell, D. (2012). Partnering for change: An innovative school-based occupational therapy service delivery model for children with developmental co-ordination disorder. *Canadian Journal of Occupational Therapy, 79*(1), 41–50. https://doi.org/10.2182/cjot.2012.79.1.6

Moore, G., Audrey, S., Barker, M., Bond, L., Bonell, C., Hardeman, W., . . . Baird, J. (2015). Process evaluation of complex interventions: Medical Research Council guidance. *British Medical Journal, 350*, h1258. https://doi.org/10.1136/bmj.h1258

Morgan, C., Novak, I., Dale, R. C., Guzzetta, A., & Badawi, N. (2014). GAME (Goals-Activity-Motor Enrichment): Protocol of a single blind randomised controlled trial of motor training, parent education and environmental enrichment for infants at high risk of cerebral palsy. *BMC Neurology, 14*(1), 203. https://doi.org/10.1186/s12883-014-0203-2

Novak, I., & Honan, I. (2019). Effectiveness of paediatric occupational therapy for children with disabilities: A systematic review. *Australian Occupational Therapy Journal, 66*(3), 258–273. https://doi.org/10.1111/1440-1630.12573

Ogourtsova, T., O'Donnell, M., De Souza Silva, W., & Majnemer, A. (2019). Health coaching for parents of children with developmental disabilities: A systematic review. *Developmental Medicine & Child Neurology, 61*, 1259–1265. https://doi.org/10.1111/dmcn.14206

Olsson, L.-E., Jakobsson Ung, E., Swedberg, K., & Ekman, I. (2013). Efficacy of person-centred care as an intervention in controlled trials: A systematic review. *Journal of Clinical Nursing, 22*(3–4), 456–465. https://doi.org/10.1111/jocn.12039

Peter, D. (2019). Is the "unmotivated" client a myth? Reconstructing human service practices. *Journal of Progressive Human Services*, 1–16. https://doi.org/10.1080/10428232.2019.1583006

Polatajko, H., Cantin, N., Amoroso, B., McKee, P., Rivard, A., Kirsh, B., . . . Lin, N. (2007). Occupation-based enablement: A practice mosaic. In E. Townsend & H. Polatajko (Eds.), *Enabling occupation II: Advancing an occupational therapy vision for health, well-being and justice through occupation* (2nd ed., pp. 177–201). Ottawa, ON: Canadian Association of Occupational Therapists.

Polatajko, H., Davis, H., Stewart, D., Cantin, N., Amoroso, B., Purdie, L., & Zimmerman, D. (2013). Specifying the domain of concern: Occupation as core. In E. Townsend & H. Polatajko (Eds.), *Enabling occupation II: Advancing an occupational therapy vision for health, wellbeing and justice through occupations* (2nd ed., pp. 13–36). Ottawa, ON: Canadian Association of Occupational Therapists.

Polatajko, H., Mandich, A., Missiuna, C., Miller, L., Macnab, J., Malloy-Miller, T., & Kinsella, E. (2001). Cognitive Orientation to Daily Occupational Performance (CO-OP): Part III: The protocol in brief. *Physical & Occupational Therapy in Pediatrics, 20*(2/3), 107–123. https://doi.org/10.1080/J006v20n02_07

Pryor, J. (2018). A few more words on person-centred rehabilitation. *Journal of the Australasian Rehabilitation Nurses Association, 21*(1), 2–4.

Rathert, C., Wyrwich, M. D., & Boren, S. A. (2013). Patient-centered care and outcomes: A systematic review of the literature. *Medical Care Research and Review, 70*(4), 351–379. https://doi.org/10.1177/1077558712465774

Reedman, S. E., Boyd, R. N., Elliott, C., & Sakzewski, L. (2017). ParticiPAte CP: A protocol of a randomised waitlist controlled trial of a motivational and behaviour change therapy intervention to increase physical activity through meaningful participation in children with cerebral palsy. *British Medical Journal Open, 7*(8), e015918. https://doi.org/10.1136/bmjopen-2017-015918

Rochford, T. (2004). Whare Tapa Wha: A Māori model of a unified theory of health. *Journal of Primary Prevention, 25*(1), 41–57. https://doi.org/10.1023/B:JOPP.0000039938.39574.9e

Rogers, C. R. (1959). *A theory of therapy, personality, and interpersonal relationships: As developed in the client-centered framework* (Vol. 3). New York: McGraw-Hill.

Rosenbaum, P. (1998). Family-centred service: A conceptual framework and research review. *Physical & Occupational Therapy in Pediatrics, 18*(1), 1–20. https://doi.org/10.1080/J006v18n01_01

Rush, D., Sheldon, M., & Hanft, B. (2003). Coaching families and colleagues: A process for collaboration in natural settings. *Infants and Young Children, 16*(1), 33–47. https://doi.org/10.1097/00001163-200301000-00005

Ryan, R. M., & Deci, E. L. (2017). *Self-determination theory: Basic psychological needs in motivation, development, and wellness*. New York: Guilford Press.

Santana, M. J., Manalili, K., Jolley, R. J., Zelinsky, S., Quan, H., & Lu, M. (2018). How to practice person-centred care: A conceptual framework. *Health Expectations, 21*(2), 429–440. https://doi.org/10.1111/hex.12640

Schwellnus, H., King, G., & Thompson, L. (2015). Client-centred coaching in the paediatric health professions: A critical scoping review. *Disability and Rehabilitation, 37*(15), 1305–1315. https://doi.org/10.3109/09638288.2014.962105

Stucki, G. (2005). International Classification of Functioning, Disability, and Health (ICF): A promising framework and classification for rehabilitation medicine. *American Journal of Physical Medicine & Rehabilitation, 84*(10), 733. https://doi.org/10.1097/01.phm.0000179521.70639.83

Taylor, E. W. (2009). Fostering transformative learning. In J. Mezirow & E. W. Taylor (Eds.), *Transformative learning in practice: Insights from community, workplace and higher education* (pp. 3–17). San Francisco, CA: Jossey-Bass.

Townsend, E., Beagan, B., Kumas-Tan, Z., Versnel, J., Iwama, M., Landry, J., . . . Brown, J. (2007). Enabling: Occupational therapy's core competencies. In E. Townsend & H. Polatajko (Eds.), *Enabling occupation II: Advancing and occupational therapy Vision for health, well-being and justice through occupation* (2nd ed., pp. 87–133). Ottawa, ON: CAOT.

Townsend, E., & Polatakjo, H. (2013). *Enabling occupation II: Advancing an occupational therapy vision for health, well-being and justice through occupation*. Ottawa, ON: Canadian Association of Occupational Therapists.

Turner-Stokes, L. (2007). Politics, policy and payment: Facilitators or barriers to person-centred rehabilitation? *Disability and Rehabilitation, 29*(20–21), 1575–1582. https://doi.org/10.1080/09638280701618851

Visser-Meily, A., Post, M., Gorter, J. W., Berlekom, S. B. V., Van Den Bos, T., & Lindeman, E. (2006). Rehabilitation of stroke patients needs a family-centred approach. *Disability and Rehabilitation, 28*(24), 1557–1561. https://doi.org/10.1080/09638280600648215

Ward, R., Reynolds, J. E., Pieterse, B., Elliott, C., Boyd, R., & Miller, L. (2019). Utilisation of coaching practices in early interventions in children at risk of developmental disability/delay: A systematic review. *Disability and Rehabilitation*, 1–22. https://doi.org/10.1080/09638288.2019.1581846

World Health Organization. (2001). *International classification of functioning, disability and health: ICF*. Geneva: World Health Organization.

World Health Organization. (2013). *How to use the ICF: A practical manual for using the International Classification of Functioning, Disability and Health (ICF)*. Geneva: WHO.

Yun, D., & Choi, J. (2019). Person-centered rehabilitation care and outcomes: A systematic literature review. *International Journal of Nursing Studies*, *93*, 74–83. https://doi.org/10.1016/j.ijnurstu.2019.02.012

Chapter 3
Implementation procedures

Fiona Graham and Jenny Ziviani

OPC is a person-centred, relational approach to working with people to enable occupational performance and social participation. Since 2017, the three domains of OPC which guide therapeutic processes have been described as Connect, Structure, and Share. In this chapter we describe the current OPC domains and the elements contained within them, illustrating key points with case examples. The focus in this chapter is on describing OPC techniques in detail and illustrating their application.

KEY MESSAGES

- OPC comprises three interacting domains of practitioner focus: Connect, Structure, and Share.
- OPC combines relational and procedural components to optimise clients' autonomous decision-making regarding their goals and actions towards reaching these goals.
- In OPC particular attention is paid to cultivating a therapeutic environment which encourages client authority, choice making, and creative problem-solving.

REFLECTIVE QUESTIONS

- After reading the overview of three OPC domains – Connect, Structure, and Share, which most closely align with how you already view your practice? Which are you curious to learn more about?
- The domain of Share is the most frequently misunderstood of the OPC domains and perhaps the most challenging to the way many

rehabilitation health professionals work. Many clinicians tell us that prior to learning OPC they thought they already shared decision-making with clients, yet they discovered that clients could lead the analysis and resolution of their situations to a far greater extent than they had anticipated. To what extent do you think you involve clients in shared decision-making? Reflect upon your current practice as you read more about OPC.

- After reading each section, note down one technique that you plan to try with a client in the following week/s. What might you need to do ahead of meeting the client to ensure you do apply it?

OVERVIEW OF THE OPC DOMAINS: CONNECT, STRUCTURE, AND SHARE

The three OPC domains of Connect, Structure, and Share are graphically represented as tiered, with each reliant on the domains sitting beneath (see Chapter 1, Figure 1.1). The Connect domain guides the practitioner to establish strong, positive, and empowering connections with clients, thereby engendering a high-trust partnership. Achieving this is foundational to the effectiveness of therapeutic techniques used within the Structure and Share domains. Connect includes the techniques of listening, empathising, and partnering.

Structure forms the second tier of OPC and includes the process-related components of the intervention. Structure is intended to guide the practitioner in the sequential arrangement of OPC techniques and the specific ways in which these are used in OPC. Structure outlines the processes of establishing valued participatory goals, collaboratively analysing performance, supporting client action, evaluating goal progress and effectiveness of strategies, and generalising effective strategies to other life situations.

The third domain, Share, forms the final tier of OPC. Share describes the use of specialist interviewing strategies to encourage and assist clients to share their knowledge and ideas that will progress them towards their goals. It also offers guidance for practitioners in ways of sharing information that maintains the client as the active agent of change. The overarching intention of the Share domain is to guide practitioners to maintain the client as the active decision-maker and change agent throughout all phases of OPC. The Share domain includes the techniques of being curious, expecting resourcefulness, asking first, prompting reflection, and facilitating the learning of principles. The hierarchical relationship between the three domains is important. Eloquent, curious questions emerging from the Share domain will help the client to progress only if the client trusts that the practitioner is genuinely curious (Connect domain) and if the questions relate to a goal that the client truly values (Structure domain).

THE FIRST DOMAIN: CONNECT

The foundational domain of OPC, Connect, describes how to create the conditions for the particular type of therapeutic relationship required for coaching (see Figure 3.1). The relationship itself is a key ingredient of OPC. The essence of an OPC relationship is to establish a strong, positive, and authentic partnership with clients, enabling them to be active agents throughout decision-making. Clients' sense of autonomy is paramount at all times and is facilitated by the quality of the developing partnership relationship. Distinct from many rehabilitation interventions, this partnership is not assumed to occur. Directives to be 'person centred' are not sufficiently detailed to create a coaching partnership, irrespective of clients' apparent level of motivation, education, or other resources.

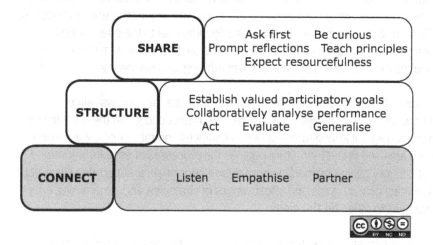

Figure 3.1 Three enabling domains of Occupational Performance Coaching, emphasising the Connect domain

Connection in OPC is successful when the client feels respected and accepted as they are, when they view the practitioner as trustworthy and as someone who understands their perspectives. Some clients may come to the therapeutic encounter assuming this type of relationship. For others this feeling of being respected and understood by health professionals may be unfamiliar. For these clients an authentic connection will only develop through considerable conscious attention and skilfulness on the part of the practitioner. The following sections provide detailed descriptions of the elements of the Connect domain: listen, empathise, and partner.

Connect: listen

All practitioners listen to their clients to some extent, but within OPC listening, specifically mindful listening, is perhaps the most powerful therapeutic technique. To listen appears deceptively simple. Listening is a skill (King et al., 2017) and as such requires attention and practice. Listening, rather than simply hearing, does not just happen because one person is talking and another is silent. Mindful listening (sometimes referred to as global listening) (Gash, 2016) is conscious, proactive, and effortful. Authentic, mindful listening results in a shared space in which the practitioner is fully attuned to the client. The client experiences this kind of listening as being validated and understood. Listening mindfully is what practitioners do during OPC in order to deepen connection, learn what goals *really* matter to clients, and appreciate what clients already know that will support their goal achievement. At a very practical level, until practitioners have listened to clients they cannot know how to apply other aspects of OPC, such as developing goals and understanding clients' existing knowledge. Listening mindfully is therefore at the heart of all other activities within OPC.

Mindful listening in OPC goes beyond active listening, as it is traditionally described (e.g., www.mindtools.com/CommSkll/ActiveListening.htm). In active listening guidance often focuses on practitioners' outward behaviours such as making eye contact, nodding, smiling, and maintaining an open posture. Attending to the outward 'signs' of listening can actually decrease the quality of listening. Sometimes, too, our intention to listen carefully to someone speaks louder than our posture (see Box 3.1). The mindful listening required in OPC shifts the emphasis to the internal activity of the listener, rather than how we are appearing from the outside.

BOX 3.1   ILLUSTRATIVE CASE. WHEN ACTIVE AND MINDFUL LISTENING DO NOT MATCH

At an OPC training workshop, Anthea was extremely nervous taking up the role of practitioner in a group role play. An experienced clinician, Anthea was anxious about 'getting it wrong' in front of the observing peers and trainer. She sat leaning forward, hands clasped tightly, frowning as she listened intently to her peer role playing a client. While mostly silent, Anthea asked questions at times to clarify or affirm something the 'client' had said and followed the client's lead on the direction of conversation. The trainer asked the pair to pause the role play to check in with Anthea on how she was going, and Anthea shared how paralysed she felt by her nerves. The trainer then asked the 'client' how it felt to be talking with Anthea. The client said she felt affirmed, 'heard', accepted, and understood and was so immersed in her own reflections that she had not noticed Anthea's nervousness. Anthea's attentive listening and genuine curiosity made a greater impression on the client than did her nervousness.

During mindful listening practitioners are simultaneously fully attuned to the emotional, sensory, visible, and non-visible messages of both themselves and their clients. To cultivate mindful listening takes practice, self-awareness, and reflection and requires development of skills in both mindful awareness and in the application of mindfulness to the task of listening.

Mindful awareness

Mindful awareness refers to knowing one's mind in this moment or 'being present' and is an important component skill of mindful listening in OPC (described previously). Mindful awareness involves awareness of our breath (e.g., is it fast, shallow, strained?); the state of our mind (e.g., are our thoughts settled, jumpy, reactive, or sluggish?); and our emotional state (e.g., are we feeling anxious, impatient, happy, or content?). It can seem a paradox to attempt to be fully mindful to another person by paying attention to our own breath, thoughts, and emotions, yet this is how we can achieve mindful listening. When we are fully aware of ourselves – in this moment – we can notice when we have become reactive to what is being said or have become distracted.

Mindful awareness while listening conveys to clients a profound acceptance (i.e., non-judgement, unconditional positive regard) of whatever is being expressed, an acceptance that this is how things are right now. Acceptance does not indicate agreement, liking, or passivity about what is discussed – simply that this is 'how it is'. Without mindful awareness our thoughts, words, actions, and emotional reactions can be directed by a desire to move away from unpleasant feelings, such as anxiety or embarrassment (Shapiro & Carlson, 2017). In the context of a rehabilitation session, this might appear as brushing over difficult things that are said or apparent. For example, a practitioner working with children with disabilities and their families, in the absence of mindful awareness, might get caught up in thoughts like:

- This would be so much easier if this family were more functional.
- I can't do much if you won't do the home programme!
- If I had a child like this I don't think I could cope as well as this mother is.
- I know I can fix this with a piece of equipment.

These kinds of thoughts would affect the practitioner's ability to listen well to the client and may influence what is said in return (e.g., convey a sense of hopelessness or impatience). Similarly a practitioner might also (unwittingly or not) avoid uncomfortable feelings by imposing rigid structures on how therapy occurs, for example by starting all new clients with a set of formal assessments so that the direction of therapy is controlled. A simple strategy to check our mindful awareness is to notice our breath, mind, or emotional state just prior to seeing a client. Observing and simply acknowledging to ourselves 'this is how it is' is a powerful way to bring our awareness into the present moment.

The challenge of listening

The challenge of listening as a health professional is not to be underestimated. Practitioners regularly comment that to 'just listen' or sit in silence with clients during OPC is their biggest hurdle. Often we fill the silence with a piece of advice, an observation, or a summary of what the client just said – all of which can diminish clients' sense of authority over their lives. Silence is important. OPC requires clients to be actively involved in reflection, problem-solving, and decision-making. Like us, they require thinking time to engage at this level; that is, they need silence. They also need us to be ready to listen (mindfully aware) when they are ready to share. One common strategy for learning to sit with silence is to count silently to ten. Alternatively try noticing ten breaths to raise your mindful awareness while you wait. Additional strategies are shared in Box 3.2.

BOX 3.2   PRACTITIONER EXERCISE. CULTIVATING MINDFUL LISTENING SKILLS

- Take a moment right now to focus your attention on your breath. You might like to close your eyes. Notice the breath rather than thinking about breathing. Notice the sensations of breathing; the chest expanding, the passing of air through your nose. Note how many breaths you can count before your attention wanders. Try doing this for a couple of minutes just before meeting a client. Notice what is different about meetings after doing this exercise.
- Another exercise to improve mindful awareness is to focus your attention on your body. Notice the muscles around the eyes, jaw, and neck. Without trying to change them, notice what happens as you simply bring your attention to one part of your body. You may like to try bringing your attention to the parts of your body in contact with ground or chair. Allow yourself to sink in to the supporting surface. Doing this in micro-moments during a session with clients can quickly anchor your attention to the present moment, allowing you to focus more fully on the client.

We become better listeners the more we can accept things as they are. We can also let go of a lot of effort and prevent the energy loss that comes from striving to make things different. We can let go of the internal conflict that sometimes arises when clients are not responding the way we might have expected or wished them to. When we focus on what simply is, right now, the expectation of there being something else drops away. During OPC, the use of non-judgemental listening is hoped to engender in clients an accurate perception that we are highly attuned to them, understanding of their circumstance, and trustworthy.

Connect: empathise

Empathy is the second element in the OPC domain of Connect. Listening involves the making of space for the client while empathy is the OPC practitioner's response to what the client does with that space. Empathy is understanding a person from their perspective rather than one's own. Many believe this is only possible through vicariously experiencing that person's feelings, perceptions, and thoughts to some extent (Empathy, 2018). It is important to distinguish empathy from a related idea, sympathy, because sympathy is much less helpful in developing coaching relationships. Sympathy is feeling pity or sorrow for someone else's misfortune (Oxford University Press, 2019). While the emotionality of the response and recognition of another's difficulty is common between sympathy and empathy, sympathy embodies a distancing from the other and usually a judgement that the sympathiser is better off in some way. This judgement conveys an unhelpful power difference between coach and client, often leading to a more distant and hierarchical relationship than is desirable for coaching.

Empathy, as described in OPC, lacks this judgement. Rather than distancing ourselves from a client's emotions (or conversely becoming swamped by these), when empathising we experience and express open-hearted, non-judgemental compassion for another's experience. Empathy lacks a moral judgement of a person's choices or perspective. Empathy requires a *recognition* of the client's emotional experience and an utter *acceptance* of how they are in this moment. This does not mean an agreement with the client but that we accept that, for the client, this is how it is right now. In relation to empathy, what the client has shared is not good or bad, serious or trivial. It simply is. The power of authentic empathy in developing connection in OPC is the trust that empathy fosters.

Empathy is a core ingredient in virtually any effective help-giving encounter and is the central mechanism for development of connection. Judging from the limited mention of empathy in most rehabilitation interventions, it is often either assumed to occur or its relevance is minimised. This is understandable when the focus of practitioners' expertise and contribution has been analysis of clients' problems and impairments, coming from a medical paradigm (see Chapter 5 for further discussion of the place of expertise). OPC in contrast comes from a strengths-based, enablement paradigm, where clients' preferences, ambitions, knowledge, and competence take precedence over expert knowledge about peoples' body structures, body functions, or other facets of their lives. It takes considerable courage for people to share their deepest fears and dreams – which we blithely probe as we ask clients what their goals are in rehabilitation. Consider how many people in your life know what really matters to you, your deepest wishes and insecurities. Consider how comfortable you would be to say these aloud to someone you just met in a multi-bed ward. The privacy of this information attests to the degree of vulnerability required to share it, and thus the importance of empathy in OPC, where the meaningfulness of goals to clients is central to its effectiveness. The more we trust a listener, the more honest we will be. Based on this trust, developed through empathy, skilful coaching conversations will kindle new insights for both client and coach.

So how do we 'do' empathy in the context of rehabilitation? Whether empathy has occurred is best judged by the client's experience of feeling validated, accepted, and understood rather than our own actions or words. But we, as health professionals, control our expression of empathy. The roles, environments, and systems in which we work as rehabilitation professionals can result in challenging circumstances in which to develop high-trust relationships and convey empathy authentically. Box 3.3 lists some specific ways in which empathy can be consciously expressed.

BOX 3.3   PRACTITIONER EXERCISE. FINDING WAYS OF CONSCIOUSLY EXPRESSING EMPATHY

- **Listen mindfully**. Ask open-ended questions that put you in the position of listening to your client's concerns, goals, current experience, and ideas. Listen mindfully to what they say. Notice and quieten your inner chatter. Focus your attention on the emotional experience of the client and the fullness of what is being expressed.
- **Notice your own emotional response to what the client expresses**. Your emotional response may be felt as tightening in the chest, a rising panic (*"Oh no, I don't have time for this"* or *"How on earth will she achieve that goal?"*). You might feel sadness and reflexive compassion for the client's story. In turn, responding compassionately to yourself about the feelings that arise in these moments allows you to be more empathic to others. The first step, however, is noticing your emotional response as it happens. For the lucky few, this self-awareness may come naturally. For many of us though (especially in our professional roles and environments), noticing requires focused attention and a re-patterning of our automatic inner dialogue. Just noticing and kindly 'sitting with' the feelings that arise is often all that is needed for the feeling to abate and allow you to experience compassion and project empathy for your client. To have an emotional response to our clients' situations is normal. But if you are routinely overwhelmed by your emotional response to clients, you might want to seek someone with whom this can be discussed. When applying OPC, emotional blocks curtail the development of connection with clients. This in turn may curtail clients' honesty, creativity, and development when with you, thus emotional self-awareness is an important prerequisite to implementing OPC.

- **Find a point of shared human experience with clients**. It may be as superficial as a place you both know, something they are wearing that you admire, a shared interest in sport, music etc.
- **Let your compassion show**. When you consciously relax your body (notice your body, adjust your posture, and choose to 'let go' of an area of tension), you will be able to express your compassion and empathy more clearly.
- **Convey empathy in words**. Less is often more in expressing empathy verbally. Try saying nothing when you next feel the compulsion to speak to a client, and then notice the effect. When you do speak, a simple but effective way to convey empathy is to simply state one or two words the client has used that hold the emotional weight of their message. In the following example, the practitioner could have chosen from any of the underlined words to echo an empathic response.

Client:	Oh gosh, I just <u>don't know where to start</u>. My <u>life is such a mess</u> at the moment. It's only three months since I split with my husband. The landlord just put the rent up so we are going to have to move again. Little Johnny's behaviour has gone nuts. He is pinching himself all the time and he is almost impossible to get to school. <u>It's all I can do</u> to keep my job and feed everyone. . . . [10 seconds silence then client's eyes well up]. I'm not sure <u>how much more of this I can take</u>.
Practitioner:	It's all you can do. . . . [silence. Client nods].

Empathy and self-care of practitioner

Attention to the emotional experience and needs of others as required in OPC can be emotionally draining and place practitioners at risk of burnout. However, in our experience of OPC, the empathic engagement is countered by the excitement and joy of seeing clients succeed. Furthermore, the mindful approach to engagement with clients proposed here has been found to reduce stress among health professionals (Burton, Burgess, Dean, Koutsopoulou, & Hugh-Jones, 2017). Attention to our emotional reserves is important for maintaining our resilience and enjoyment of our work. See Box 3.4 for some ideas for maintaining our own wellbeing. Some people think of this as refilling their empathy tank.

BOX 3.4 PRACTITIONER EXERCISE. FINDING WAYS OF FUELLING UP THE EMPATHY TANK

Share the good, hilarious, and triumphant experiences as well as the hard times. Take a mindful moment and let these really sink in. While respecting client privacy and confidentiality, share the joys with colleagues to fill up the whole team.

- Focus on your compassion for clients' experiences rather than projecting an outer image of empathy. Projecting takes more emotional energy than simply recognising and accepting clients' emotional experiences.
- Remind yourself that the emotions and events shared by clients are not *your* experiences. Notice your emotional state, tone, and body after discussions that required a lot of compassion and empathy, and mindfully let those experiences go as you depart the meeting. Some people find it useful to imagine putting the feelings on a leaf and watching them float away.
- Move your body. A walk, swim, dance, sport, or yoga session in which we have an intense physical experience is a good way of resetting the mind and body and letting go of residual feelings that belong to a session and not with us.
- Time in nature (or listening to nature sounds) is also known to help to calm and reset the mind (Capaldi, Passmore, Nisbet, Zelenski, & Dopko, 2015). Where is a good place or time that you could bring this into your week/day if you find you are holding on to clients' experiences beyond your meetings with them?
- Consider taking up a regular meditation practice. There are many forms of meditation, including non-secular meditation traditions, groups, and courses.

Empathy is expressed authentically and used therapeutically in OPC to help meet clients' need for connection (thereby building trust). Clients differ in their need for empathy, and this is likely to fluctuate over the course of one coaching relationship (usually there is a greater need in the early stages of relationship building) or even the course of one session. We, as coaches and practitioners, also have differing levels of need for connection. It is important that our expression of empathy be based on the client's need for connection, rather than the practitioner's need (Taylor, 2008). An important reflection for the practitioner is 'how much empathy is helpful here to facilitate change for *this* client?' While this is an abstract judgement, a cue from clients that the intensity of empathy should reduce is a sense of recoiling from the practitioner or dismissal of practitioners' attempts to convey empathy.

Connect: partner

Partner is the final element in the OPC Connect domain. Partner describes practitioners' intention to foster a power-neutral relationship with the client, in order to maintain, or in some cases enhance, the client's position as the active agent of change. The practitioner begins cultivating a partnership in OPC from the first contact with a client. First, through listening mindfully and empathising with the client, the practitioner establishes the conditions for a power-neutral partnership. However, enacting a partnership also requires explicit actions of power sharing with clients, including sharing authority for decision-making and recognition of mutual expertise.

Partnership relationships have long been advocated in the person-centred and family-centred literature as described in Chapter 2. From the perspective of disability/consumer rights, there is the argument that clients have the right to direct their own healthcare; from the perspective of health behaviour change, there is also the argument that people are more likely to adopt and sustain new behaviours when they experience a high sense of autonomy in choosing those behaviours (Deci & Ryan, 1987). OPC aligns with both of these arguments in the inclusion of partnering as an important quality of therapeutic relationships. While partnering with clients can seem simple and an obvious approach, actually doing this in many health settings can be difficult and require very conscious efforts by the health professional. These efforts are critical to effective use of OPC.

Why is partnering challenging?

Partnership relationships are challenging to develop in healthcare settings – particularly in inpatient settings where the medical model tends to dominate (Crom, Paap, Wijma, Dijkstra, & Pool, 2019). Some have argued that true partnership relationships are not possible in a help-seeker/help-giver relationship (Gzil et al., 2007) with many factors contributing to a complex power dynamic. When health professionals are in gatekeeper roles, where they hold responsibility for tasks such as approving funding for adaptive equipment or carer support, a sense of equal partnership may be undermined. Time pressure, real or imagined, creates an impetus to be task-oriented and efficient, which may come at the expense of partnership with clients, as we subtly or overtly rush conversations, make decisions for clients, or curtail the options available to clients. Healthcare systems are notoriously hierarchical, with expertise being a key indicator of status, and we therefore often feel the need to present as 'experts' to our colleagues. Clients also sometimes expect us to be 'the expert', to be authoritative and to effectively solve their problems. However, when targeting change in occupational performance and participation in life roles, the clients' expertise of themselves and their contexts becomes critical to goal progression.

When coaching we need to be cognisant of the psychological processes at play which may prompt clients to view the health professional as the expert with all the answers. This could be, for example, a reflection of grief and adaptation in the face of lifelong changes in their (or their loved ones') health condition. Such changes usually require adaptations and active engagement by clients in how these are enacted (Novak, Morgan, McNamara, & Te Velde, 2019). In OPC we actively draw clients' attention to their own expertise (perceptiveness, insight, observations, wisdom) to develop partnerships in which clients' authority over their lives is emphasised. Negotiating the sharing of our expertise is permissible in OPC but is minimised and secondary to seeking out clients' expertise (see Share domain later in this chapter for further explanation of sharing information with clients).

Have we got time to partner?

Practitioners working from an expert-based paradigm often raise a concern that it takes too much time to allow clients to reflect and make choices, with many commenting, *"We've seen clients in similar situations, many times before so we know what they need to do. Coaching just takes more time to reach the same conclusion"*. In contrast, practitioners who have switched from an expert-directed approach to OPC have commented that coaching *saves* time in the longer term (see Chapter 6). The time from first meeting to solution does take longer with OPC than an expert, practitioner-directed approach. However, time is often saved in the long run through multiple mechanisms: Client engagement is heightened as goals become more specific to clients' priorities, thus clients are more likely to enact strategies. Clients also often want to see the practitioner less frequently as they take greater responsibility for enacting plans and determining if plans are working, and clients often terminate therapy before the maximal allowed number of sessions are reached. While we don't advocate OPC as a strategy to minimise client contact, we suggest that the slower initial pace required when partnering with clients is often at least made up for over the course of intervention. An economic analysis of OPC compared to usual care is currently underway (Graham et al., 2019) which will help clarify the impact of OPC on therapist time and resources.

How can we cultivate partnership?

Achieving partnerships with clients in most rehabilitation settings will require a conscious effort by the practitioner. Our choice of words, the way we position our bodies, the activities we do with clients, and the formality of dress can all convey our status in the relationship – as the expert or as a collaborative partner. While it can be helpful to note these external cues of power/status, as with mindful listening, when we have an intention to engage with clients on an equal footing the gestures indicating partnership tend to follow.

Even asking a client what time or place would be convenient to meet subtly positions clients as active decision-makers. Each opportunity for the client to make a decision or share an opinion solidifies their self-perception as an active and equal partner in the therapeutic relationship (see Box 3.5).

BOX 3.5   PRACTITIONER EXERCISE. EXPLORING SPECIFIC WAYS TO CULTIVATE PARTNERSHIPS DURING OPC

- Physically positioning yourself at eye level with the client – sit alongside if they are sitting/lying down.
- Avoid a barrier between you and the client, such as a desk.
- Minimise note taking in front of the client unless strictly essential.
- Frame things as 'we' rather than I/you, such as *"We are going to work together on this"* and *"When you are ready we can take a look at how your arm is working and what we can do to help it along"*. Write down some phrases in your own words that convey partnership rather than expertise.
- Avoid a preamble about your expertise when introducing yourself. Instead, link your role to the clients' goals if these are known, e.g., *"Hi I'm Sally the OT and I'm here to help with your goal to get back home"*. Rehearse your own introduction that conveys partnership with clients.
- Consider the implication of status in your choice of clothing, make-up, shaking hands. Does it helpfully position you alongside your clients or does it signal a divide?

- Avoid summarising what clients have said (summing things up in your own words) as this emphasises power differences. Instead convey curiosity and naivety, and ask permission to check if you have understood correctly. Use paraphrasing that draws on the very words the client used, as in the earlier example of expressing empathy. Experienced coaches use fewer words to paraphrase (de Jong & Kim Berg, 2008).

 Before continuing reading, this might be a valuable place to take a break to reflect on the ideas presented in the OPC Connect domain before moving on to the second of the three domains of OPC: Structure.

THE SECOND DOMAIN: STRUCTURE

The Structure domain provides the framework and temporal sequence of OPC through which the practitioner guides conversation, sitting above Connect in the three enabling domains of OPC (see Figure 3.2). Structure in OPC is a problem-solving process that includes processes of goal setting, performance analysis, action, evaluation, and generalisation of effective strategies. Each of these steps is common to many interventions, however the way each step is undertaken in OPC is specific and their combination is unique. An overarching feature of

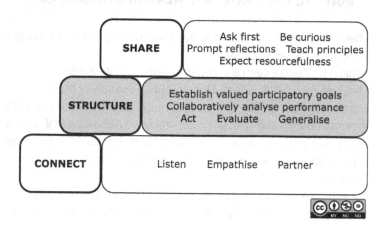

Figure 3.2 Three enabling domains of Occupational Performance Coaching, emphasising the Structure domain

the structured problem-solving process used in OPC is the situating of agency with the client. Goals are wholly clients' goals (not practitioners'). Analysis of situations occurs through exploring clients' (rather than therapists') perception of how things are occurring. Action refers to clients' actions to affect progress towards their goals. Clients, rather than practitioners, evaluate the extent to which progress is made. Clients decide if and how successful strategies can be generalised. Hence, within OPC the process is described using the specific terminology of (1) establish valued participatory goals, (2) collaboratively analyse performance, (3) act, (4) evaluate, and (5) generalise. The following section describes each step in detail, with examples of how each can be applied using different clinical scenarios.

Structure: establish valued participatory goals

Goal setting is widely considered best practice in rehabilitation (Brewer, Pollock, & Wright, 2014; Kolehmainen et al., 2012; Levack et al., 2006; McPherson, Kayes, & Kersten, 2014), but it is described in quite diverse ways (Levack, Dean, Mcpherson, & Siegert, 2006a). Here, we describe how goal setting occurs in OPC, particularly in the positioning of agency with the client.

Goal setting in OPC involves a conversation with the client to identify the way of 'being in the world' that the client aspires to for themselves and, when appropriate, their child, other loved one, or family. Within OPC, goal setting is considered *part of* the coaching, rather than a preliminary step to the 'real work' of therapy. Often, it is the goal clarification itself which facilitates clients' insights and ultimately promotes change. Goal setting is the first step in OPC because knowing what clients value and prioritise informs all subsequent coaching.

Clients may not know the language of goals, but everyone has an opinion on what is most important to them right now (D. Kessler, personal communication, 12 July 2019). Therefore, a classic question posed by practitioners to start a conversation about goals in OPC is *"What matters most to you right now?"* Gaining a clear understanding of the client's goal usually requires several cycles of communication, with the practitioner seeking clarification about what that future (achieved goal) state might look like and asking questions to resolve any ambiguity in the client's description. The importance of the goal to clients is paramount, hence the practitioner explicitly asks clarifying questions and looks for signals (e.g., verbal emphasis, repetition, emotionality) that indicate what is most meaningful to the client in their goal description.

Why do goals need to be 'valued'?

The more deeply the client values the goal, the more amplified is the clients' goal striving (Locke & Latham, 1984). Goals in rehabilitation generally are used for multiple purposes, including to identify clients' priorities, organise teamwork, evaluate practitioners or services, and access funding for the service (Levack, Dean, Siegert, & Mcpherson, 2006b). In OPC, goals are principally used to identify client priorities and support client autonomy by explicitly linking goals with planned or intended actions by the client. Although goal achievement is also used in research to evaluate the effectiveness of OPC, clients' valuing of their goals is paramount.

Valuing of a goal is only reflected in the meaningfulness (McPherson et al., 2014) that the person being coached attributes to the goal. During OPC clients' valuing of goals is identified by listening for cues as to what part of a situation matters most and what meaning it holds. It is often *not helpful* to directly ask 'why' questions, such as *"Why does that matter to you?"*, because these questions lead people to hypothesise (think) rather than reflect (feel), and it is the feeling that is the clue to what matters most.

Cues to what matters most might be given in the client's tone of voice, for example conveying more emotion with some words than other words. Values might also be indicated as clients describe two seemingly contradictory goals or actions. Respectfully asking for clarity around these contradictions can help us to understand an underlying value that unifies both goals, and makes one a priority, thus revealing which is more deeply valued. Empathy coupled with goal-directed action is a powerful combination for change. In Box 3.6 Fiona shares her reflections on a case that highlighted the influence of client values on the direction of therapy when using OPC.

BOX 3.6   PRACTITIONER REFLECTION. THE POWER OF VALUES IN OPC

I was working with the mother of an eight-year-old boy with developmental co-ordination disorder (DCD), who wanted her son to manage his cutlery better. After a couple of coaching sessions the mother described that she didn't really care about her son's cutlery use. It was the tantrums he had when he couldn't do things, and the way she felt manipulated by him, that really bothered her, because she feared he would grow up to be a selfish, wilful young man. Despite the departure from direct functional effects of DCD, the occupational restrictions of these issues was within my scope of responsibility as an occupational therapist. I applied OPC with the mother to explore her aspirations for her son.

To clarify her current goal, I asked her what kind of young man she wanted her son to grow into, to which she responded, *"A good man, who is respectful, who has good friends. Someone I enjoy the company of"*. While the mother didn't explicitly state it, it seemed that she valued respect, self-control, and social connection a lot more deeply than she did fine motor skills. To understand how these values could be expressed in occupational/participatory terms, we talked through what her vision of 'a good man' would look like when he was the age her son was currently, and she immediately linked addressing of her son's reaction to challenges in the daily routine (including frustration with cutlery) to the skills she wanted her future son to have. Her commitment to this vision enabled her to overcome difficult feelings (shame, incompetence) when she tried to assert herself with him and she quickly progressed with her goal on cutlery use, as well as several other aspects of the daily routine. In this example of OPC, the core therapeutic process was assisting this mother to identify what she valued most for her son.

Why do goals need to be 'participatory'?

Goals in OPC are expressed in a way that reflects occupational performance (Law & Barker-Dunbar, 2007) and participation (World Health Organization, 2001) in valued life roles, and the activities that are meaningful to clients within those roles. While debate continues as to how occupational performance and participation are operationalised in clinical practice (Chien, Rodger, Copley, & Skorka, 2014; Imms et al., 2016), very specific guidance on the wording of 'participatory goals' in OPC is given here.

In OPC, goals are defined in a 'goal statement' which include *a subject* (i.e., the client or their loved one), *an activity* (i.e., performance of an action or task) that is directly linked to a valued role, and *the social context* in which the activity meaningfully occurs (e.g., home, school, work, or elsewhere in the community). Goals also include an indication of the *extent* of occupational performance and participation (e.g., how often, how much, or how intently) (Imms et al., 2017; Randall & McEwen, 2000). Several examples of OPC goals are provided in Table 3.1. Further examples of participatory goals are provided in Appendix C and a tool to guide OPC goal development, in Appendix D.

Table 3.1 Examples of occupational performance and participation goals appropriate to OPC

Goal statements: In each of these goal statements, the subject is indicated by name, the activity is in italics, and context is in bold
Toby *asks for help when stuck during play* **at preschool**.
Theo *shares attention on a toy* **with mum**.
Meisha *chooses play activities* 3 times per day **at kindy**.
Alice *resolves conflict when playing* with her sister **at home**.
Angie attends ***dance classes*** weekly.
Steve undertakes paid *work,* **onsite**, 20 hours each week.
David *cooks dinner* **at home** independently twice a week.
Alisha and her three (disabled) children *travel* **internationally** within the next six months.

The precise wording of an OPC goal that reflects valued participation-focused change very much depends on the client and their context. Consequently, OPC goal activities will vary in complexity from brushing teeth independently to attending school/work to successful international travel. This is consistent with suggestions that participation occurs on a continuum from simple to complex (Kolehmainen et al., 2019).

Context is important in participatory goals because all meaningful, sustained change in occupational performance and participation occurs somewhere in clients' lived environments. It is only when change occurs 'in the real world' that progress is considered to be made in OPC. Specifying the context in OPC also acknowledges that solutions often lie in the context itself and may only work in that context. In another context, different or modified strategies to achieve the same activity may be needed. When the goal activity occurs in multiple contexts, it is a helpful coaching strategy to encourage clients to think about one context at a time and to identify which context they wish to start with, knowing that some transference of successful strategies to other contexts is likely to occur. Broadly, most real-world contexts are covered by the descriptors of 'home', 'school', 'work', and 'in the community', although more specific descriptors such as 'during soccer practice' or 'in the playground' will be more appropriate for some goals.

A goal of a person completing an activity in the clinic or with the practitioner would *not* be appropriate for OPC because change in this context does not necessarily reflect meaningful change in the context of a person's life roles. Similarly, a goal to achieve change in a skill or task performance in the person's lived environment but only with the practitioner (e.g., in practitioner-child play at the preschool) would not be an appropriate goal or indicator of goal achievement in OPC because this level of change does not reflect a difference in the person's social roles, such as being a playmate or student. Practice of a strategy with the practitioner (under ideal conditions) might be valuable in refining the strategy, but this rehearsal is never the goal in OPC because it does not reflect a change in occupational performance and participation in the lived environment. A notes page and blank template for developing goal statements with clients is provided in Appendix D.

How do we describe degree of change or the scale of OPC goals?

In OPC the focus of the goal needs to be personally meaningful to clients, as does the *degree of change*. For example, a parent might have a goal for their child to get ready for school independently. For some parents this goal might only be meaningfully achieved when the child needs no verbal prompting. For another parent one verbal prompt per task might be considered a significant and meaningful improvement. Sometimes clients describe a level of change that we, as practitioners, think is easily achievable. At other times clients propose goals that seem highly ambitious. Often practitioners worry that clients will choose *overly* ambitious goals if permitted to dictate the degree of improvement or scope of the goal. In our experience this seldom happens.

If goals need to be what the health professional might consider 'ambitious' in order to be meaningful to the client, then meaningfulness takes precedence. Rather than feeling concerned about encouraging 'false hope', the practitioner using OPC remembers that:

- When people are striving for what is most meaningful to them they invest considerable effort and attention.
- When working towards participation-focused goals endless solutions are possible, making it very difficult to predict outcomes for individual clients (in other words, anything is possible).
- In OPC clients are also the agents of change and evaluators of progress, thus the client (rather than the practitioner) reviews the balance of effort and progress at each coaching session, and their appraisal may differ from that of the practitioner.
- To clarify the degree of change desired from a client's current performance to goal achievement, the practitioner might ask the client to reflect on the

following: What are the indications that they (or their loved one) are ready to achieve the goal? What is the timeframe over which they would like to work on this goal? What is the degree of change they would expect or hope for within this timeframe?

How can we measure goal progress?

Documenting goals and goal progress is a requirement of OPC. Goals, worded according to the template provided in Appendix D, are ideally documented within the first OPC session. Because goal setting itself is considered a part of the therapeutic process of OPC, goals can change over sequential coaching sessions, as clients gain insights into their motivations, actions, and circumstances. However, clients' original goal statements are still reviewed at the end of an episode of care, even if additional goals are also added during the course of intervention. While this can be challenging when using goal attainment as an outcome measure, the focus of OPC discussions remains on what is most meaningful to clients.

It is recommended that goal progress be formally evaluated in clinical and research use of OPC. To date, research on OPC has used the Canadian Occupational Performance Measure (COPM: Law et al., 2005) and/or Goal Attainment Scaling (GAS: Kiresuk & Sherman, 1968) to formally measure goal progress because these measures accommodate the priorities of individual clients and have well-established psychometric properties for a range of health populations (Carpenter, Baker, & Tyldesley, 2001; Carswell et al., 2004; Cup, Scholte op Reimer, Thijssen, & van Kuyk-Minis, 2003; McDougall & Wright, 2009; Steenbeek, Ketelaar, Lindeman, Galama, & Gorter, 2010; Tennant, 2007). Information about the relative merits and overlap between COPM and GAS are discussed elsewhere (Calder, Ward, Jones, Johnston, & Claessen, 2018; Cusick, McIntyre, Novak, Lannin, & Lowe, 2006). Based on preliminary studies of OPC, only one of the two measures is necessary for research purposes (Graham, Rodger, & Ziviani, 2013) because the direction and degree of change measured is consistent between the measures.

Both COPM and GAS require the drafting of an individualised statement that is then either rated or assigned a position on a scale. When using either the GAS or COPM in OPC, it is important that the client goal is documented with limited interference from the practitioner (e.g., as per earlier descriptions of coaching, the practitioner does not attempt to temper or extend the scale of the goal to be more 'realistic' or less 'ambitious').

The COPM historically measures 'problems' rather than goals. In OPC the COPM is modified to document and measure *goals*, i.e., aspired future states, rather than *problems*. Consistent with the solution-focused coaching perspective of OPC, there is a substantial difference between goals and problems as discussed throughout this chapter. The practitioner does not go systematically through all domains of self-care, productivity, and leisure to identify problems in the way that the COPM was originally designed to be used (Law et al., 2005). Instead the practitioner asks what is *most important* to the client (rather than asking for perceived *problems*) as this relates to self-care, productivity, and/or leisure, and documents this in the appropriate place on the COPM form.

Whose goals are targeted in OPC?

The subject at the focus of goals in OPC is an important ethical question, as the subject is not always the person being coached. Caregivers (including parents, teachers, paid caregivers, and spouses) of people with disabilities may have legitimate concerns and needs in relation to their charges. OPC was originally developed for and is often used with caregivers (e.g., parents, spouses, or teachers) of people with disabilities who may reasonably seek coaching to achieve goals related to someone else's actions. This might occur when the client cares for someone who lacks insight into a situation for which a goal may be in their best interests. For example, a parent of a ten-year-old child with developmental co-ordination disorder may reasonably have a goal that their child be able to get ready for school independently, as achieving this goal is an important life skill in many cultures. The husband of a woman with a significant brain injury may seek help to achieve the goal that his wife can go shopping without squealing loudly or banging her head when she gets excited. Both of these goal examples would be appropriate to OPC when the subject of the goal also values a related outcome. For example, the ten-year-old would also like to be less dependent on his parents in the mornings (or at least have them 'nag him' less); the head-injured wife enjoys shopping and could go more often when the squealing and head banging are minimised.

Whenever possible, the subject of the goal should be included in determining the goal during OPC. When the goal subject and the caregiver are both present at coaching, the practitioner can pose the coaching questions to both parties, accommodating the communication level of the person with the disability. In some situations it may not be appropriate for the person with a disability/child to be present for the coaching conversation, but their perspective may be important to clarify the goal. In this case the person being coached might make a plan to seek the opinion of the goal subject – in whatever way is appropriate to their communication level – and discuss this information with the practitioner the following week.

Even when the person with a disability cannot participate in a coaching conversation about goals that relate to them, their motivation and preferences surrounding the goal are an important consideration in identifying solutions toward goal achievement. When the subject of the goal clearly communicates that they do not wish to be taking part in the goal activity, then this needs to be openly discussed with the client. It is unethical and inconsistent with OPC principles (such as person-centredness) to assist clients towards goals that the subject of the goal has no interest in pursuing. Further guidance in clarifying the motivation of the person with a disability is provided below as part of the broader process of collaborative performance analysis.

Sometimes clients identify goals over which they have limited influence. For example, a goal that 'a child is invited on playdates' is challenging given that achieving this goal depends on the decisions of other families. A client having a goal about returning to driving after a stroke despite vision and motor impairment and compulsory loss of license is similarly problematic because legal vision requirements will prohibit the client from ever driving. These situations need to be handled carefully during OPC in order to maintain partnership with clients and avoid the practitioner 'having the final say' in which goals are permissible (Kessler, Walker, Sauve-Schenk, & Egan, 2019). A balance needs to be struck between supporting client autonomy (e.g., the right to have highly ambitious goals and to hold on to hope for a desired future) alongside honesty with clients in sharing professional information critical to goal outcomes.

One strategy to maintain the meaningfulness of goals when the practitioner knows a goal is impossible (such as returning to driving after a severe stroke) is to ask the client what the achievement of this goal will enable them to have or do that is ultimately why this goal is so important. For example, the adult with stroke may say that driving a car allows them to be independent or to keep in touch with family. Two goals can then be drafted: one about returning to driving (with a view to re-evaluating the value of this goal and progress toward it at each session) alongside a second goal around being in contact with family regularly – a goal which has many possibilities as to how it is achieved, such as learning to videoconference or use public transport.

What does OPC with multiple clients look like?

In keeping with person- and family-centred practice, OPC has been successfully undertaken with single or multiple clients present. Combinations of clients have included one or two parents (or caregivers, including teachers), with or without their children/dependents present and involved in coaching conversations.

Involvement of all stakeholders in determining the direction of therapy that relates to them is desirable from both human rights (Rutherford Turnbull III, Beegle, & Stowe, 2001) and behaviour change perspectives (Michie, van Stralen, & West, 2011). While the presence or absence of multiple clients, particularly dependents, during coaching has been proposed as a delineating factor in types of coaching (Ogourtsova, O'Donnell, De Souza Silva, & Majnemer, 2019), this has not arisen as a barrier to application of OPC or a determining factor in its effectiveness. In contrast, flexibility about clients' decision to include or exclude significant others in OPC is one of the advantages of OPC.

While involvement of multiple clients in coaching conversations in OPC demands a greater level of skill by the practitioner, the same OPC intervention principles apply of identifying a shared, valued goal and client(s)-led identification of strategies believed to realise goal visions. Involvement of multiple clients can manifest as seeking the contribution of multiple parties to the framing of goals, as well as in identifying ways to achieve goals. If agreement on a goal cannot be reached, or if there are also individual-specific goals in addition to shared goals, the practitioner may coach clients separately.

The main challenge in coaching multiple clients together is in arriving at a genuinely shared goal. Arriving at a shared goal involves giving each client an opportunity to express their preference for how they want things to be and minimising venting of problems or blaming of others. The practitioner's skill in maintaining non-judgemental and empathic engagement with all clients concurrently will underpin each clients' honesty and ability to then move on to considering solutions.

An observed effect of OPC when multiple clients are coached is that a more collaborative interaction style is taken by the client with their co-clients and other stakeholders in goal progress (Graham, Rodger & Ziviani, 2016). When all key stakeholders in a life situation have a clear goal to which they are committed, goal progress tends to be faster than with only one stakeholder involved.

The presence of children/dependents who may be the subject of goals at OPC sessions requires careful consideration. In some instances their presence offers the advantage of in vivo coaching through performance analysis and strategy development (e.g., experimenting with positioning to improve self-feeding at mealtimes). Children/dependents may also be present purely due to limited caregiving alternatives. At times the presence of children/dependents is unhelpful, as the parent/caregiver may need to express thoughts or feelings that are not helpful or healthy for the child/dependent to hear. In OPC the practitioner poses the question of who would it be helpful to have present to the client, revisiting this decision as circumstances change.

In the case example in Box 3.7, OPC is undertaken with the parent only and then child and parent together to achieve one goal. The practitioner extends the goal-setting conversation beyond the mother's initial concern to identify the child's concern in the same situation. The appropriateness of the child's presence is negotiated throughout the episode of care resulting in the decision that she is present some of the time and absent at other times.

BOX 3.7   ILLUSTRATIVE CASE. OPC CAN ACCOMMODATE MULTIPLE CLIENTS: A CASE EXAMPLE OF OPC WITH A PARENT AND A CHILD WITH NEURO-DISABILITY

Trish, the mother of an 11-year-old girl (Jas), approached Alice, an occupational therapist in private practice for help to minimise Jas's frequent emotional outbursts. Using OPC, Alice and Trish arrived at the goal for Jas to go to bed before or at the same time as the other family members. Currently, Jas woke the rest of the family as she went to bed at midnight, and Trish wondered if the lack of sleep contributed to Jas's outbursts and difficulty with mornings. Trish had already tried a lot of things and had concluded that Jas found it very hard to express herself and just did not seem to care about getting to sleep or her impact on the family. At this stage the goal was clearly Trish's but the subject of the goal was Jas. Alice suggested that Jas attend the next session with Trish. Using the F-words (function, family, fitness, fun, friends, and future) (Rosenbaum & Gorter, 2012) to focus Jas's attention on what she would like to be different, Alice guided Jas to articulate her goal, which ultimately became for everyone to stop nagging her to go to bed earlier (among other things). Alice used the COPM to clarify Trish's and Jas's perspectives on how this situation felt before they began addressing it with OPC (see Box 3.7). Trish and Jas shared this goal despite it being founded in differing motivations and having differing levels of importance.

Within the same session, Alice asked Trish and Jas how they would like the bedtime routine to look. Jas wanted to be independent and not nagged at, but she also wanted everyone to be happy with her. She could see that if she went to bed earlier it would be better, but she wanted to go when she wanted. Trish wanted to be able to get to sleep herself and know that her

Table 3.2 Trish and Jas's pre-intervention COPM scores

Goal	Importance /10		Performance /10		Satisfaction /10	
	Trish	Jas	Trish	Jas	Trish	Jas
For everyone to stop nagging me to go to bed earlier	10	2	2	6	1	3

daughter was getting enough sleep. They made a plan together for Jas to set an alarm at 8.30pm to get her bag ready for school the next day, and then she would get ready for bed. She would set a second alarm to be in bed by 10pm. The next week they rated this goal in terms of performance and Trish scored 7, while Jas scored 8, both significant clinical improvements.

Alice continued to coach Trish alone in subsequent sessions around supporting Jas to overcome other issues like screaming at mealtimes. Alice remained open to the idea that Jas may attend another session in future, but for now, Trish wanted to develop her own skills in supporting her daughter.

On reflection, Alice commented that she felt Jas's involvement in the OPC session was critical to achieving this outcome. In Alice's words, *"many times, without engagement from the child even the best strategies won't work"*. Alice recognised that her therapeutic effect for this mother and daughter was in large part the development of a shared goal in which both of their voices were heard.

Structure: collaborative performance analysis

Collaborative performance analysis (CPA) is the phase during OPC when new ways of going about goal situations are most closely envisioned and explored with clients. Like all aspects of OPC, agency as to how this process unfolds and what changes or strategies are explored sits with clients. The practitioner asks questions that guide clients' analysis of the goal situation rather than asking questions to aid their own analysis. The practitioners' role is to guide clients through the iterative process of analysis, reflection, and decision-making.

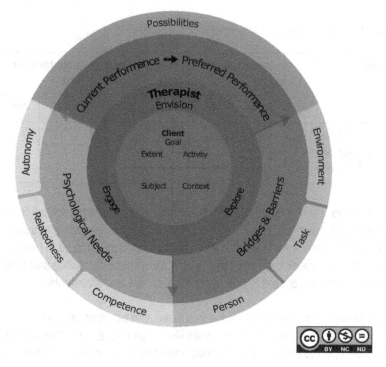

Figure 3.3 Collaborative performance analysis and its relationship to goals within Occupational Performance Coaching

Source: Figure 1.1 Three enabling domains of Occupational Performance Coaching. First published Graham, F. (2020), Occupational Performance Coaching Resources. Retrieved from www.otago.ac.nz/opc (29/01/2020). This work is licensed under a Creative Commons Attribution-NonCommercial-NoDerivatives 4.0 International License. University of Otago. Reprinted with permission.

The CPA process is illustrated in Figure 3.3 represented by the outer three rings. The inner circle reflects the goals already established upon which CPA discussion occurs. The practitioner's questioning guides the client in (1) *envisioning* possibilities for the preferred performance; (2) *exploring* bridges (facilitators) and barriers to make the goal a reality; and (3) *engaging* in analysis and decision-making. Ultimately, the practitioner coaches the client to identify and implement a few small, targeted actions that the client perceives will move them closer to goal achievement.

Collaborative performance analysis: envision

CPA begins with the practitioner guiding clients to *envision* how they want things to be. Often clients want to start by relaying what currently happens (current performance) or what they wish was *not* happening (e.g., that I am not in pain;

that my child does not have meltdowns). Having already identified clients' broad goals in the first phase of the Structure domain, the practitioner prompts the client to describe in more detail how they would prefer a situation to be (preferred performance). The conversation focuses on the unconstrained possibilities for how things could be, rather than restricting the vision to what is immediately solvable or absolutely achievable. Ambitious visions are often the most engaging for clients. The practitioner directs the conversation to how the client wants things to be, even if the client returns to describing the problem. Exploration of solutions in OPC is heavily weighted towards analysis of the achieved goal rather than analysis of the current problem. This difference is more than semantics. An orientation to solutions rather than problems makes a profound difference to the strategies identified and the extent of change observed (Grant & Gerrard, 2019), although how the vision is described by the client will vary. Clients may describe the physical or social setting, their own or their child/dependents actions, or the emotional tone of a situation (i.e., what would *feel* different when the problem has gone away). All of these qualities clarify to the client and practitioner what the most meaningful future state is, but not all qualities need to be covered to develop this shared understanding.

During the envision phase, a couple of things often happen. Clients can be preoccupied with the current problem and continually redirect conversation back to the problem. The practitioner's role here is to respectfully acknowledge the clients experiences and perceptions of the problem, but instead reorient the conversation to clarifying what the client wants the situation to look like. A practitioner can start to feel frustrated, mirroring the client's own experience of frustration. Practitioners' mindful awareness of their own state is really important in order to respond (rather than react) in ways that are useful to the client. In order to envision an alternative way for challenging situations to resolve, the client needs to make several cognitive shifts. Psychologically, the client needs to accept what is unchangeable (e.g., their/ their dependent's health condition) and consider that their response to it could be different. It takes a degree of self-confidence and self-compassion to do this, as well as trust in the practitioner. The practitioner's demonstration of patience, kindness, and commitment to the emerging vision becoming a reality provides an important model for clients stuck in the current 'problem' mind-set.

The following transcript (Box 3.8) illustrates a coaching dialogue in which the client is stuck in describing the current (problem) situation. The practitioner has to be persistent in respectfully reorienting the client to how they want things to be, related to a parent's goal of her son, Gabriel, getting ready for school independently. The kind of questioning by the practitioner is sometimes referred to as 'the miracle question', however the word miracle does not need to be used (de Jong & Kim Berg, 2008). The client response that is intended through orienting the client to solutions is that the client creates a mental picture of what it looks like when the goal is achieved and shares this with the practitioner.

BOX 3.8 ILLUSTRATIVE CASE. A COACHING EXAMPLE WHEN A CLIENT IS STUCK IN A 'PROBLEM' MIND-SET

Practitioner: If you rolled all the good days you've had into one fantastic morning, talk me through what happens as Gabriel gets ready for school really well.

Client: He probably had a really good night's sleep. I try to get the kids into bed by 7.30 but it often goes on until 8. They often want to watch something extra on TV and then Gabriel needs to do some reading, so it gets pretty late sometimes by the time he gets to sleep.

Practitioner: So on this morning that he got ready for school really well, he was in bed by about 7.30 and had a really good night's sleep. He wakes up in the morning and he's in a pretty good mood . . . Then what happens?

Client: I think he'd just come down stairs, at about 6 or 6.30. Rather than me having to call him he would just come down and ask 'what's for breakie?' He seems to be in a better mood when he comes down by himself. Jackson [younger brother] might have slept in so it's just Gabriel. Because when they both get up together they start playing and distract each other. It's quite variable who gets up first normally.

Practitioner: Right. And on this day that he is getting ready for school really well Gabriel is up first on his own and he asks 'what's for breakie', then what happens?

Client: Well he starts having his breakfast, and he eats it fairly quickly. You know, he isn't playing with his toys or reading something instead of eating.

One common consequence of the envisioning phase of CPA is that the client becomes emotional while describing their vision of how they want life to be. The emotion may be expressed as tears of sadness, a raised angry voice, or intense laughter. The emotion is often an indication of a psychological shift occurring – the transition from feeling stuck to feeling that there are possibilities for a better way of living. Again, this is an important point for the practitioner to notice her own emotional response and to remain emotionally available to the client. If the practitioner withdraws from the client's emotionality (i.e., shuts down internally), most clients will pick up on this subconsciously and put their own emotional guard up, restricting a transition to a solutions-focused and possibilities mind-set.

Often, the envisioning conversation will be as enlightening for the client as it is to the practitioner, particularly when the client has felt 'stuck with the problem' for some time. Once the client's vision is clear, the practitioner and client are then ready to explore the bridges and barriers to making the vision a reality.

Collaborative performance analysis: explore

Exploring bridges and barriers, like the rest of OPC, is done with the client in the driver's seat with a focus on possibilities and solutions (rather than problems or impairments). The explore phase involves drilling down into the details of what exactly the situation will be like, when the problem is absent or alleviated, so that the client can identify changes that they perceive as likely to work. The explore component of CPA is a form of task analysis, a core skill of occupational therapy and some other rehabilitation professions. It is beyond the scope of this manual to provide detailed instruction on task analysis, as this is considered a prerequisite skill for OPC (see Chapter 4). Distinctively, in OPC performance analysis is led by clients rather than the practitioners and incorporates clients' psychological needs within the analysis itself. Like the envision phase, there is not a checklist of things to cover because the possibilities of what might be relevant to finding solutions are endless. Most of the time, the direction of analysis questioning is guided by clients' previous statements about what they think might help improve goal performance. Attempting to cover too many avenues for solutions also limits the potential for clients' reflection and development of insight. The depth of detail explored will evolve over the course of intervention and depends on how specific the analysis is to identify the next steps for change.

It is common that bridges and barriers will only tentatively be explored in the first OPC session, with the majority of time being dedicated to envisioning and goal setting. In subsequent OPC sessions, the explore phase integrates the new knowledge gained as strategies have been tried. The practitioner questions the client about the effects they observed these changes had on the goal situation and the client's views on how well performance now matches their initial vision.

During the explore phase of CPA, the practitioner follows the client's lead on the possibilities discussed, with the onus on client's development of insight, rather than detailing of facts. Often a single core insight (with associated behaviour changes) is all that is required for clients to achieve their goals, consistent with transformational learning experiences (Mezirow & Taylor, 2009). Adding more detailed analysis or trying to prompt multiple insights can detract from the momentum of one substantive realisation. To explore bridges and barriers, the practitioner may initially ask general questions like:

- *What have you found helps?*
- *When do things tend to go better (or worse)?*
- *What do you know about your health condition/your child for handling this situation well?*
- *What supports you as you try to make this happen?*

As clients share information about what happens when they attempt the strategies they have identified, practitioners' questions become more specific. Like the narrowing of a funnel, exploratory questioning in OPC often goes from general to more specific aspects of the goal situation.

The PEO model (Law et al., 1996, described in Chapter 2) offers a conceptual framework for practitioners to use while guiding clients in exploring bridges, barriers, and solutions to their goals. The PEO prompts conversations about the client ('person'), the context in which the goal is based ('environment'), and the specific tasks involved (elements of the 'occupation'). Each of these avenues for exploration are discussed in more detail in the next sections.

Several practitioners have reported to us that they share the OPC process graphic, which incorporates the PEO (see Appendix B) with clients when using OPC, and find it supports clients in reconsidering where solutions may lie. When there is a good match between the task demands, the client's abilities, and environmental supports, the client can most readily go about living their vision, and that is the primary objective of OPC. The phrase 'make it match' is used to remind practitioner and client that there is no hierarchy in where solutions come from – person-, task-, and environment-based strategies are of equal value.

EXPLORING THE 'PERSON'

Key aspects of the person (who is the subject of the goal) to consider are their (1) *motivation* to complete the task, (2) *knowledge* about the task, and (3) *ability* to do the task.

When the goal is about a child or dependent, often the person being coached has made assumptions about what the subject wants or knows. Motivation is a complex phenomenon, and low motivation from either the client or the goal subject needs to be probed further in OPC. Questioning around the client's and subject's experience of autonomy, relatedness, and competence in the specific performance context of the goal often highlights unmet psychological needs which can be addressed once identified.

A common comment from parents involved in coaching is *"But we've done this routine a thousand times – my son must know what is expected!"* – only to learn, after asking her son what he knows, that he has a wildly different idea of his mother's expectations. Early action plans during OPC are often to investigate the knowledge and motivation of key players in goal achievement in more detail, by simply asking them.

Discussion of the steps of performance may also reveal that the goal subject does not currently have the ability to complete the task in the way that the client expects, and therefore alternative approaches to the task can be explored. Ideally the question-reflection cycle enables clients to reach these conclusions independently. Sometimes clients need time to observe the situation more closely (e.g., between sessions), thus the 'plan' for the week may simply be to 'observe'. Alternatively, the practitioner may offer to share information about teaching and learning principles such as grading tasks, facilitated learning, or errorless practice (Graham, Sinnott, Snell, Martin, & Freeman, 2013; Greber, Ziviani, & Rodger, 2007; Jones et al., 1996) to enable the client to consider alternate routes to success, being careful to place agency for decision-making on that information with the client.

EXPLORING THE 'TASK'

Consideration of the (1) number or sequence of steps and the (2) expected standard of the task can elucidate bridges or barriers to goal achievement. As clients describe differences between what currently happens and how they want situations to be, the practitioner listens for and prompts clients to explore additional steps in the task or alternative sequences of steps which could bridge these gaps. For example, a parent may describe that the child transitions from play to meal times more easily when given verbal notice two minutes before changing tasks. The practitioner could guide the parent to explore use of this strategy during other transitions. Questioning clients to explore the specific standard of task performance, such as level of independence, speed of completion, or quality of outcome, are valuable avenues to solutions. Sometimes simply raising our expectations of ourselves or others prompts improved performance (e.g., raising the expectation that children put toys away when finished playing supports progress on a goal of self-management in getting ready for school). Conversely, lowering expectations of the quality of performance can support goal progress. For example, high expectations of weightlifting performance while attending the gym can be a barrier to achieving a goal of regularly attending the gym.

EXPLORING THE 'ENVIRONMENT'

Often the changes that enable clients to progress towards goals lie in the immediate physical or social environment of goal situations. Parents and caregivers can be a part of a child's or dependent's social environment while also being the person engaging in coaching. Dimensions of the environment that a practitioner might explore with the client include proximity, intensity, complexity, and consistency of the environment. For example, a person may be more successful in a goal situation when help is closer at hand or, conversely, farther away (proximity). Cues may be more effective when intense (e.g., loud, bright) or when more subtle. A complex environment (such as a bustling coffee shop) compared to a simple one (e.g., a library) might improve or curtail performance. As in all aspects of OPC, when thinking about the environment in which performance occurs, practitioners' role is to prompt clients' reflection, analysis, and decision-making about strategies rather than determine the appropriate solution.

Collaborative performance analysis: engage

Engagement is a core element of collaborative performance analysis, referring specifically to clients' engagement in the process of analysing goal situations and making change in their lives. As in the Connect domain of OPC, the three basic psychological needs of self-determination theory – autonomy, relatedness, and competence (ARC) – guide practitioners' thinking (see Chapter 2). We posit that within CPA when clients' psychological needs are met, they are better able to choose and apply strategies that are congruent with their values and life circumstances. Client autonomy is addressed as the practitioner poses questions which explore goals highly valued by the client. Practitioners foster clients' sense of relatedness by indicating respect for clients' perspectives and commitment to supporting achievement of their goals. Clients' sense of competence (ability and confidence in abilities) is enhanced by questions and prompts that encourage clients to describe examples of their coping, resourcefulness, creativity, and persistence. Specific examples of the ways a practitioner might attend to these psychological needs to optimise client engagement during the performance analysis process are provided in Table 3.3.

Table 3.3 Examples of attending to psychological needs for autonomy, relatedness, and competence during collaborative performance analysis

Psychological needs	Collaborative performance analysis steps	Practitioner questions and prompts
Autonomy	Envisioning	*Can I clarify with you, is it getting more artwork completed that is important for you, doing art with others, or something else?*
Autonomy	Explore: Act	*We've talked about a couple of ideas for getting your son to sleep through the night, Susan. What are your thoughts at this point about supporting your son with sleeping?*
Autonomy	Explore: Person	*With what you know about your energy and strength since your stroke, how long a shopping trip do you think you could manage at the moment?*
Autonomy	Explore: Task	*Can you talk me through it, step by step: what do you need to do to get breakfast ready at your house?*
Autonomy	Explore: Environment	*How is the play space arranged when baby Timmy moves his body more during play? How many toys would be out?*
Relatedness (understanding)	Explore: (person, task, or environment)	[in response to a client's reflection] *That makes sense to me, Dave, especially given your experiences with your boss.*
Relatedness (trusted)	Explore: (person, task, or environment)	*I can hear your frustration Alice. You have tried a lot of things to get your son to bed.*
Competence (confidence)	Explore: task-action	*When you imagine using that idea of 'just letting your son play with his food', does it feel doable? How confident are you feeling about setting up some food play and leaving him to it?*
Competence (outcomes)	Explore: task-action	*When you imagine using that idea of 'just letting your son play with his food', what do you see yourself doing while he is playing? OR Is there anything else you feel you need to do to be able to use this transfer technique on your own?*

Structure: act

Act reminds us that OPC is not just a friendly chat. Change towards achievement of clients' goals requires the client doing something differently. Act comprises two parts: First, the client's stated intended action, and second, actually doing it.

Act: intentions

Simplicity is the key to action statements that lead to action. Small changes are preferable to large or complex changes, as the former are more likely to be carried out and sustained. The practitioner guides clients to consider what feels manageable and what they are confident will work. Often the phrases *"Does this plan feel doable to you?"* And *"How confident are you that this is likely to work?"* are used to explicitly clarify these points. It is always better to know sooner than later if a client does not intend to carry out a plan or is unconvinced that it will work. Often these questions lead to a refining of the action plan. Sometimes a client's only action might be to observe a specified situation more closely for a few days. This kind of action plan is preferable to a plan that won't be carried out and will result in a sense of failure for the client. Simply observing is often also a powerful way for clients to enhance their sense of competence (thus becoming more ready to act) through gaining insight into a situation.

The practitioner guides clients to describe a strategy in their own words, even if the main strategy is a specific technique that you have just explained (see Box 3.9). It is important not to change their wording in any summarising of the plan unless they have grossly misunderstood some information that was shared by the practitioner. Clients are more likely to do as *they* said and less likely to act if we have imposed ownership on an idea by rewording it.

BOX 3.9   PRACTITIONER EXERCISE. KEEP THE 'FIVE SS TO ACT' IN MIND WHEN COACHING CLIENTS TO CHOOSE ACTIONS

- Keep it *small*. Big change often starts with small steps. Big steps often don't happen.
- Keep It *simple*: Just 1–3 simply stated actions within plans.
- Let clients *state* and confirm the planned actions in their own words.
- A *snowball effect* often occurs from small initial steps. Be patient and trust the client's lead, including allowing them to learn from mistakes.

- Real (lasting) change *sticks*. Actions that didn't fit the client or context will not be sustained so need to be refined or abandoned, without judgement.

Act: doing it

Sometimes clients report back that they implemented the plan discussed last session and "voila", it worked! Celebrate these easy wins but don't expect them often. More often clients report an unforeseen barrier when they attempted the plan – perhaps a lack of confidence within themselves or a reaction from a family member that they did not expect. Other times, clients have taken themselves through several cycles of analysing performance, acting, and evaluating by the time we see them again and their plan now looks very different from the one that was last discussed. All of these scenarios are 'grist for the mill'; important information to coach more deeply into enduring strategies, embedded in clients' lives. Concepts such as 'non-compliance' and 'non-adherence' are not relevant in OPC since the plan was owned by the client rather than imposed or prescribed by the practitioner. Non-action by a client is viewed as very valuable information for further CPA. Whether the planned action has occurred or not, coaching returns to the CPA process, centred around goal achievement, exploring bridges and barriers but incorporating this new information based on clients' observations.

Structure: evaluate

Evaluation occurs after a plan is actioned. This might be within one session, for example after a technique (e.g., an altered body position or new piece of equipment) has been attempted. Evaluation also happens at the beginning of every subsequent coaching session, with the client initially evaluating their own progress. The practitioner asks, *"How are you doing with [description of goal] now?"*

Evaluation comprises two main elements: (1) evaluation of progress towards the goal and (2) evaluation of how effectively the plan worked. Typically, the practitioner first explores performance of the goal. Has anything changed from the client's perspective? Any change (large or small, positive or negative) is of interest because this indicates to the client that change is possible and that the client can be an agent of change. Change is always framed as positive progress because it means we have learnt something more about the situation that we can use to develop more refined strategies. Other questions the practitioner might ask to guide client's evaluation of progress include:

- *What have you noticed about [goal activity] this week?*
- *What happened during [goal activity] the time it went best?*
- *What happened on the worst day this week?*

The practitioner might also use scaling questions (Greenberg, Ganshorn, & Danilkewich, 2001) to guide the client to quantify their evaluation more specifically. Scaling questions go something like this: *"On a scale from one to ten, with ten being great and one being terrible, how would you rate performance over this past week?"* Or, *"If this situation was one step better (or worse), what would it look like instead?"* It is common for people to forget where they started from and to recalibrate the current performance as the 'new bad day'. Scaling questions are a good way to help clients keep a track of how far they have come and to be more specific in their observations of change. Asking clients to describe performance at one or two steps in the scale worse than and better than their current rating of performance also helps to make progress, and next steps, more explicit because clients visualise change occurring as they describe it.

The second element of evaluate in OPC is evaluating the effectiveness of the plan. The practitioner will explore through questioning, did the plan work? Does the client perceive that the plan worked? Did only part of the plan work, therefore does it need refining? This is the point within OPC where very context-specific conditions can be uncovered that are hugely influential on the success of a plan. Factors such as other members of the household, the attitude of the sports coach, the width of the aisles at the supermarket, or bus timetables can emerge as barriers to otherwise plausible strategies. Personal factors can also be revealed as influencing the success of action plans, such as a mother's cultural values around children's independence. Here, 'evaluate' segues back into a deeper layer of collaborative performance analysis.

Client agency takes precedence in the evaluation phase as in other phases of OPC. It is the client who determines progress towards the goal rather than the practitioner. Although the practitioner may offer her/his opinion as a way of reframing clients' evaluations, it is ultimately the client who decides if a plan is working and if progress is being made. The rationale for this is based on the highly person-centred philosophy of OPC, but at a pragmatic level, a client's future actions and choices will be based on what they perceive works, rather than what a practitioner or other believes.

Structure: generalise

The final step of Structure in OPC is 'generalise'. Generalise is a point where the practitioner explicitly prompts the client to consider where else a successful strategy could be used – in different contexts, with different tasks, or at different times. By successful strategy, we mean a strategy that the *client* has identified as successful in pursuit of their goal in their life circumstances.

Encouraging a client to think about the core principle of a strategy makes the strategy more readily generalisable. For example, a client with post-concussion syndrome might identify that they can manage their shopping more successfully when they plan out their trip before they leave the house. The core principle here could be 'plan ahead' or 'write the plan'. The practitioner might prompt generalisation by asking, *"Where else might it be useful to plan ahead?"* Other common examples include taking my time; one step at a time; get ready (mentally or physically); keep it calm (or take a breath) (Graham, Rodger, Ziviani, & Jones, 2016). Sometimes clients identify a metaphor or mantra for the key principle, which can be a powerful memory aid, e.g., 'smell the flowers' as a cue to take a deep breath when feeling overwhelmed.

Key areas to prompt generalisation include other settings where the task occurs; other people who support the subject of the goal to do a similar task; other times of day; and other tasks or life roles such as student, worker, or parent. Often a strategy can be relevant in multiple situations with little or no modification. However, clients may benefit from prompting to anticipate how a successful strategy might need to be modified to work into the future, especially if a developing child, recovery process, or evolving situation is involved.

Question prompts could be:

- *Who else could benefit from knowing about this strategy you discovered?*
- *What is really important for this person (e.g., teacher aide, paid carer, partner) to know to be able to use this strategy as well as it is working for you?*
- *What other tasks do you do with Johnny where this idea of 'one thing at a time' might be helpful?*
- *When you think about the daily/weekly routine, when else is it helpful to 'keep calm'?*

- *If you were to use this strategy at work/home (other context), how might it look?*
- *What might this strategy look like when your son is six months/three years older? How might it need to be modified?*

The Structure domain outlines an iterative process from identifying goals through to generalising successful solutions. Guided by this process, the practitioner asks targeted questions that prompt client reflection and decision-making, enabling clients to lead the discovery of solutions and attribute progress towards goals to themselves. The final enabling domain of OPC, Share, outlines how practitioners facilitate client-led learning.

 Before continuing reading, this might be a valuable place to take a break to reflect on the ideas presented in the OPC Structure domain before moving on to the third and final domain of OPC: Share

THE THIRD DOMAIN: SHARE

The Share domain of OPC guides practitioners in positioning clients as adult, self-determining learners while practitioners are facilitators of clients' learning (see Figure 3.5). Sharing knowledge in this way can feel strange for many practitioners who may see their role as knowledge holders (or experts) about clients, their health conditions, or their circumstances. Some practitioners have described a sense of feeling lost about where their 'expertise' lies when they find they are no longer imparting the expert knowledge traditionally held within their profession (Graham, 2018; Litchfield & MacDougall, 2002). Yet, shifting the exchange of information in therapy, to an emphasis on *clients'* sharing of knowledge, has its advantages. Clients' sense of competence and autonomy are amplified when clients realise how much they already know about how to achieve their goals. Conversely, clients are significantly less likely to enact change when they are informed, advised what to do, or prescribed solutions (Apodaca et al., 2016). Through CPA, progress towards goals of improved life situations often comes down to simple, everyday choices and actions (e.g., getting up 30 minutes earlier; asking a colleague for help; changing the seating plan at the dinner table). The practitioners' skilfulness (or expertise) becomes more centrally about *how* they engage with clients to elicit knowledge and maintaining client agency rather than *what* practitioners know about them. How to engage with clients during OPC is reflected in both an attitude of the practitioner and through some specific actions. Share components sit atop Connect and Structure domains as without these preceding elements, the techniques within Share are unlikely to be received with effect by clients (see Figure 3.4).

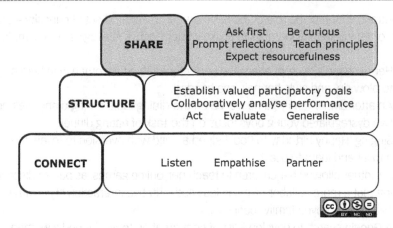

Figure 3.4 Three enabling domains of Occupational Performance Coaching, emphasising the Share domain

Source: Figure 1.1 Three enabling domains of Occupational Performance Coaching. First published Graham, F. (2020), Occupational Performance Coaching Resources. Retrieved from www.otago.ac.nz/opc (29/01/2020). This work is licensed under a Creative Commons Attribution-NonCommercial-NoDerivatives 4.0 International License. University of Otago. Reprinted with permission.

Share: curiosity

When practitioners adopt an attitude of curiosity during OPC, clients are encouraged to share their knowledge. For some practitioners this idea may seem naïve, even wasteful of time, but the effect is often that very creative solutions and powerful change emerge for clients. A curious mind-set is a signature feature of solution-focused approaches (de Shazer, 1984) (of which OPC is included). Some practitioners trained in OPC have used the term 'curious questions' to describe the open-minded, curious approach with which they interact with clients. This is characterised by a practitioner wondering, *What unique set of circumstances will this client orchestrate to realise their own success?* A curious mind-set contrasts markedly with an 'expert mind-set', which may lead to the trap of thinking, *I've seen it all before. I know what's needed here.* Practitioners trying to following the edicts of OPC outlined so far may also hear an inner voice stating, *now I just have to wait until the client figures it out.* With an 'expert' mind-set and a tendency to over-estimate the value of familiarity with common client issues, we can start to feel bored or impatient when trying to implement client-led analysis of OPC, and clients are likely to pick up on this. The expert stance will subtly restrict our ability to guide clients' exploration of possible solutions.

In contrast, adopting the role of the naïve enquirer – a mind-set of curiosity – takes us on often fascinating journeys to unlikely but effective strategies, for example:

- Her husband's microphone stand perfectly enabled a woman with hemiplegia to blow dry and style her hair, one handed.
- An after-dinner family game placed on the dining table during dinner helped two dysregulated young boys focus on the task of eating dinner.
- Singing 'Happy birthday to Poo' helped a child with aversion to toilets to sit on a toilet and learn to use it.
- A mother allowed her children to teach her online games, as part of discovering that a more collaborative and less authoritative interaction style with her children improved family routines.
- A Google search to develop a list of conversation topics helped a woman expand her ways of starting conversations and making new friends.

Other phrases used to explain and encourage a curious mind-set include practicing 'not knowing' (de Jong & Kim Berg, 2008). As with the adage, 'don't think of a pink elephant', it is difficult to imagine alternative ways of achieving goals when a fixed idea is already held in the mind. It's often necessary to consciously remind ourselves that we don't know what the solution will be in order to 'un-train' ourselves from engaging in problem-solving while a client is talking. Thinking of the character role that we adopt when coaching can also help us choose our mind-set. The Socratic role of 'naïve enquirer' can be useful here. While we do know a lot as rehabilitation practitioners, we really don't know what is going to work for this client, in their context, at this time, so some naivety is certainly justified. A curious mind-set keeps our questioning open and reinforces to clients with authenticity that they are the ultimate knowledge holders.

Share: expect resourcefulness

Alongside a mind-set of curiosity, it is helpful to hold an expectancy of clients as resourceful and capable. This is consistent with the concept of autonomy (Deci & Ryan, 1985) but is mentioned here in relation to learning transactions within OPC as a reminder that it applies to all clients being coached, at all stages of recovery. Clients know their circumstances best and the resources that they can draw upon in pursuit of goals, which are not always obvious to the client or practitioner. When we expect (rather than doubt) that a client will find a way forward with their goal, we are more likely to pause that bit longer to allow time to reflect, to pose another curious question rather than give up on the client and provide advice. More strategically, asking clients how they have managed to cope or how they keep going despite the difficulties can be effective in eliciting resourcefulness. While clients are sometimes living in very restrictive situations, our belief in their capability is an important foundation in enabling them to draw fully on what they have available.

Two strategies to encourage client sharing in OPC are to 'Ask first' and 'Prompt reflection'. Both of these strategies position clients as the experts while guiding them toward goal success.

Share: ask first

Asking a question before offering advice or a clinical opinion or stating an observation immediately places the client in control of finding solutions. It is important to avoid sounding like an interrogator (e.g., with a series of quick-fire questions) or patronising (e.g., by seeking a particular answer) when posing questions. The curious and expectant mind-set described previously helps avoid these scenarios. Similarly, the mindful listening skills described in relation to the Connect domain also prompt the practitioner to ask first, before passing comment or offering information. A conscious awareness of the pace of questioning also helps – fast enough that the client keeps their mind on the goal, but slow enough to allow space for reflection.

Simple strategies to optimise client autonomy and knowledge sharing are to ask open-ended questions (Murray et al., 2019). Specifically, questions starting with how, if, what, when, or who encourage reflective, exploratory responses while drawing attention to remembering or imagining actions related to the goal situation. The open-ended questions best avoided are those starting with 'why'. These tend to draw clients into theorising or interpreting the meaning of events, moving away from conversations about their actual experience and the concrete evidence of what actually works in their life context.

Often our professional training and experience leads us into analyst mode, and at times during OPC specialist rehabilitation, knowledge may be an important component of identifying solutions. Within OPC, however, the practitioner explores client knowledge first and only shares their own knowledge when a relevant knowledge gap for the client is clearly identified. Practitioner knowledge can be thought of as tools in the practitioner toolbox. In OPC, the toolbox is left at the door, until (if at all) it is really needed. Our experience with OPC suggests the toolbox of practitioner knowledge is needed a lot less often than we have previously assumed. An '80:20 rule' can be applied to remind us that the balance of attention (80%) should be on working to elicit client sharing of *their* knowledge, with only 20% or less attention on what we, as practitioners, share.

Table 3.4 contrasts examples of statements that could be made by a practitioner with an expert mind-set with an OPC alternative, in which the practitioner's focus is on situating agency with the client.

Table 3.4 Practitioner responses which reflect agency situated with clients: Examples of what this might sound like in OPC

Non-OPC: Agency situated with the practitioner	OPC: Agency situated with clients
That isn't a realistic goal in my experience.	What is most important for you about . . . getting back to work/your child learning to talk?
It's important that we take things one step at a time.	What would the first step look like for you?
There are quite a lot of developmental steps before your son will be able to walk.	What have you noticed your son is challenged by at the moment, but having some success with?
Your daughter seems to be what we call a 'sensory seeker'. There are specific types of activities that can help her to be more settled.	What have you noticed about the kinds of sensations your daughter enjoys? When does she enjoy these in ways that help her to focus on her play for longer?
This is a really common situation. I have a handout of tips on how to manage it – here you go.	Tell me more about how you have learnt to manage this situation. What else have you considered trying?
Visual schedules can really help in these situations. Have you tried these already?	What have you noticed about when things have gone really well? What kinds of strategies does your son seem to respond well to?
This is not something that you can manage on your own, Alice.	Who else can support you with this, Alice?
I'll need to do a full assessment before I'll know exactly what is happening here.	What is your hunch about what is going on for you?
Consistency is really important for kids, as I'm sure you know.	When you think of times that things have gone better than usual, what was different?

Share: prompt reflections

Reflection is an abstract process that involves giving deeper than usual consideration of something (reflection, n.d.). In contrast to a 'passing thought', reflection is often associated with insight – an altered awareness or understanding of a situation. In order to encourage reflection in OPC, the practitioner poses questions that (a) prompt a deeper consideration of a situation and (b) prompt the client to think of a situation from a different perspective than they normally would.

The open-ended how, if, what, when, and who questions described in Table 3.4 are an important starting point for encouraging the client to give a situation deeper consideration. The pace of questioning is also instrumental to reflection. A sufficiently slow pace of questioning will encourage a client to slow down and allow their thoughts to move beyond surface levels.

Clients may be helped to gain a fresh perspective if they are asked what they would do if they met this sort of problem in a different life role, particularly one in which they have a higher sense of competence that they do at the moment. For example if a client is seeking coaching in her role as a parent and finding it difficult to keep calm when her child has a tantrum, asking what she would do to keep a cool head when things get tense at work might remind her of some basic self-regulation strategies that she has already used effectively (e.g., take a breath, step back etc.).

Prompting clients to reflect on a situation from the viewpoint of another person can also help. It might be helpful to ask clients to imagine what they would think was a reasonable course of action if they saw someone else in their situation (e.g., a teacher, a work colleague, a family member, or a stranger). Observing bystanders such as the cat, dog, or a fly on the wall can add lightness to reflections and avoid perceptions of judgement that can come from human roles.

Prompting reflection from different time points can also lead clients to gain insights and be a way to situate new knowledge with clients. For example, the practitioner might ask, *"What do you know now about this situation that the younger you (or 5-, 10-, 20-year-old you) didn't have the benefit of knowing?"* *"When you imagine the wise 80-year-old you, looking back on all your efforts right now, what would she want you to know?"* More immediately, reflection can be prompted by asking what is different between how things are now and how they were six months ago; or what will need to be done differently as things progress, say in two years' time.

For some clients, reflection will need to be very concrete, for example immediately after a strategy has been attempted in the session. For other clients, reflection can be more abstract, but as OPC is concerned with clients' occupational performance and participation in life situations, the focus of reflections is on performance and participation in life contexts and life situations.

Share: teach principles

OPC emphasises uncovering and building on what clients already know to facilitate progress toward goal achievement. However, a critical piece of information, unknown to the client, can sometimes accelerate progress. It is not the intention within OPC that clients discover everything for themselves, but giving direct advice (e.g., *"You should . . ." "What's needed here is . . ."*) is avoided. Information provision without active engagement of the client is contrary to OPC. As the practitioner shares information, there is a risk that clients' sense of their own expertise and authority is diminished. To minimise this, practitioners first consider, *Is it clear that there is a gap in the client's knowledge in this area, or do I need to ask another question to clarify what they know about this topic or strategy? Does the information that I am thinking of relate explicitly to the goal the client identified? Does the client need to know this information at this time, and do they think they need to know it?* More information to the client doesn't always mean more power when it comes to doing things differently in everyday life. Too much information can be overwhelming and detract from the client's readiness to take action. In OPC, information is only presented that:

- Relates directly to clients' goals.
- Builds on information that the client has already expressed (i.e., what they already know).
- Links directly to decisions about action that could be taken.

In OPC we are mindful that one-sided delivery of information by the practitioner, with no expectation of client contribution to that information, encourages passivity (or learned helplessness). Hence, the *type* of information given and the *way* information is presented in OPC specifically creates opportunities for clients' active engagement in the information exchange. In OPC the content of information shared by a practitioner focuses on principles and concepts rather specific instruction or advice. The practitioner might, for example, explain the concept of self-regulation as it applies to keeping calm or focused when learning a new skill. Metaphors, such as a thermometer or simple graph, can be helpful ways to make the principle more concrete, without telling the client what they should do or recommending a specific technique. The word 'recommend' is not appropriate to OPC because it situates knowledge so strongly with the health professional.

Instead, the practitioner might state, *"Some families/clients have found X idea useful. Is this something you are interested to hear more about?"* In written reports, alternative headings to 'Recommendations' could be 'Agreed Plan' or 'Client Identified Strategies/Actions'. Similarly, principles of learning or task analysis might be shared by the practitioner, such as only changing *one thing at a time* or *identify the steps* without explicitly stating what step should be done.

The 'info club' illustrated as a club sandwich (see Figure 3.5) is a helpful metaphor to understand how information can be shared by practitioners in OPC in a way that upholds clients' agency. The outer bread represents clients making active decisions about if or what information is shared, while the fillings represent information that the practitioner imparts. First, the practitioner asks the client if they would be interested to hear about an idea or information that could be helpful – for example, she might say, *"What you are describing reminds me of the idea that strategies*

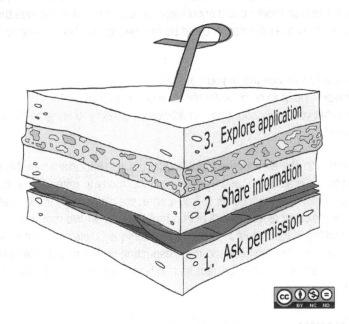

Figure 3.5 Occupational Performance Coaching 'info club' process for sharing information with clients. Permission to share information is asked first, followed by provision of information if the client assents. Finally, clients are asked if and how they envision applying the information.

Source: Figure 1.1 Three enabling domains of Occupational Performance Coaching. First published Graham, F. (2020), Occupational Performance Coaching Resources. Retrieved from www.otago.ac.nz/opc (29/01/2020). This work is licensed under a Creative Commons Attribution-NonCommercial-NoDerivatives 4.0 International License. University of Otago. Reprinted with permission.

work differently depending on our stress, or arousal levels. Would you like me to explain what I mean?" This invitation to choose if information will be shared can be subtle (noticing cues that the client is interested in deciding to expand on the explanation) or more overtly stated, as in this example. But the principle, that it is the client who gives permission – i.e., actively chooses for the information to be imparted – reinforces the client's agency. Next, the practitioner briefly shares the information directly related to the goal, represented by the centre slice of bread. They might briefly explain how arousal levels vary for everyone and affect the way we experience things, or explain a disease process that is influencing the client's experience. Information is kept brief and explicitly linked to the client's goal.

The final outer bread represents an invitation to the client to reject, apply, or build on the information. Again, this might be overtly asking the client, *"When you think of your situation, how could this idea apply?"* or might be simply pausing to allow the client to reflect and comment. A significant point here is that the practitioner is open to the client rejecting the relevance of the information entirely or making it their own. The practitioner could encourage the client to make the idea their own by asking how the information could be tailored to the client's situation, for example:

- *What would that look like in your family?*
- *What would need to be done for this to work at your place?*
- *Given what you know about your child/boss, how do you imagine this idea working?*

When information shared with the client is rejected, it is important that this is welcomed by the practitioner and used as an opportunity to reiterate clients' good judgement. It is always better to know what the client really thinks than to assume that the client agrees or will act on the information. We may indeed be wrong in thinking that some information or a technique is relevant, or it may be the wrong time for the client to hear about it. Respecting the client's choice to receive information or act on it is an important step in both client and practitioner moving forward in finding solutions.

CONCLUSION

In this chapter the OPC domains of Connect, Structure, and Share, and their respective elements, have been detailed. The development of strong therapeutic partnerships, client-led goal setting and situation analysis, and ways of sharing information between client and practitioner are described, linked by a prioritising of client-held agency for the direction of coaching conversations. The following chapter outlines processes for ensuring that each domain is applied with fidelity to descriptions in this chapter for clinical and research applications.

REFERENCES

Apodaca, T. R., Jackson, K. M., Borsari, B., Magill, M., Longabaugh, R., Mastroleo, N. R., & Barnett, N. P. (2016). Which individual therapist behaviors elicit client change talk and sustain talk in Motivational Interviewing? *Journal of Substance Abuse Treatment, 61*, 60–65. https://doi.org/10.1016/j.jsat.2015.09.001

Brewer, K., Pollock, N., & Wright, F. V. (2014). Addressing the challenges of collaborative goal setting with children and their families. *Physical & Occupational Therapy in Pediatrics, 34*(2), 138–152. https://doi.org/10.3109/01942638.2013.794187

Burton, A., Burgess, C., Dean, S., Koutsopoulou, G. Z., & Hugh-Jones, S. (2017). How effective are mindfulness-based interventions for reducing stress among healthcare professionals? A systematic review and meta-analysis. *Stress and Health, 33*(1), 3–13. https://doi.org/10.1002/smi.2673

Calder, S., Ward, R., Jones, M., Johnston, J., & Claessen, M. (2018). The uses of outcome measures within multidisciplinary early childhood intervention services: A systematic review. *Disability and Rehabilitation, 40*(22), 2599–2622. https://doi.org/10.1080/09638288.2017.1353144

Capaldi, C. A., Passmore, H.-A., Nisbet, E. K., Zelenski, J. M., & Dopko, R. L. (2015). Flourishing in nature: A review of the benefits of connecting with nature and its application as a wellbeing intervention. *International Journal of Wellbeing, 5*(4). https://doi.org/10.5502/ijw.v5i4.449

Carpenter, L., Baker, G. A., & Tyldesley, B. (2001). The use of the Canadian Occupational Performance Measure as an outcome of a pain management program. *Canadian Journal of Occupational Therapy, 68*(1), 16–22. https://doi.org/10.1177/000841740106800102

Carswell, A., McColl, M. A., Baptiste, S., Law, M., Polatajko, H., & Pollock, N. (2004). The Canadian Occupational Performance Measure: A research and clinical literature review. *Canadian Journal of Occupational Therapy, 71*(4), 210–222. https://doi.org/10.1177/000841740407100406

Chien, C. W., Rodger, S., Copley, J., & Skorka, K. (2014). Comparative content review of children's participation measures using the international classification of functioning, disability and health-children and youth. *Archives of Physical Medicine and Rehabilitation, 95*(1), 141–152. https://doi.org/10.1016/j.apmr.2013.06.027

Crom, A., Paap, D., Wijma, A., Dijkstra, P. U., & Pool, G. (2019). Between the lines: A qualitative phenomenological analysis of the therapeutic alliance in pediatric physical therapy. *Physical & Occupational Therapy in Pediatrics*, 1–14. https://doi.org/10.1080/01942638.2019.1610138

Cup, E. H., Scholte op Reimer, W., Thijssen, M. C., & van Kuyk-Minis, M. (2003). Reliability and validity of the Canadian Occupational Performance Measure in stroke patients. *Clinical Rehabilitation, 17*(4), 402–409. https://doi.org/10.1191/0269215503cr635oa

Cusick, A., McIntyre, S., Novak, I., Lannin, N., & Lowe, K. (2006). A comparison of Goal Attainment Scaling and the Canadian Occupational Performance Measure for paediatric rehabilitation research. *Pediatric Rehabilitation, 9*(2), 149–157. https://doi.org/10.1080/13638490500235581

Deci, E. L., & Ryan, R. M. (1985). *Intrinsic motivation and self-determination in human behavior.* New York: Plenum.

Deci, E. L., & Ryan, R. M. (1987). The support of autonomy and the control of behavior. *Journal of Personality and Social Psychology*, *53*(6), 1024–1037. https://doi.org/10.1037/0022-3514.53.6.1024

de Jong, P., & Kim Berg, I. (2008). *Interviewing for solutions* (3rd ed.). Belmont, CA: Thomson Brooks/Cole.

de Shazer, S. (1984). *Keys to solutions in brief therapy*. New York: Norton.

Empathy. (2018). *APA dictionary of psychology*. Retrieved from https://dictionary.apa.org/empathy

Gash, J. (2016). What does the coaching conversation look like? In W. Pentland, J. Isaacs-Young, J. Gash, & A. Heinz (Eds.), *Enabling positive change: Coaching conversations in occupational therapy* (pp. 43–56). Ottawa, ON: Canadian Association of Occupational Therapists.

Graham, F. (2018). *Sadie Philcox Memorial Lecture: Coaching in occupational therapy and other rehabilitation professions – The art and the evidence*. Lecture presented at the School of Health and Rehabilitation Sciences at The University of Queensland, Brisbane.

Graham, F., Rodger, S., & Ziviani, J. (2013). Effectiveness of Occupational Performance Coaching in improving children's and mothers' performance and mothers' self-competence. *American Journal of Occupational Therapy*, *67*(1), 10–18. https://doi.org/10.5014/ajot.2013.004648

Graham, F., Rodger, S., Ziviani, J., & Jones, V. (2016). Strategies identified as effective by mothers during Occupational Performance Coaching. *Physical & Occupational Therapy in Pediatrics*, *36*(3), 247–259. https://doi.org/10.3109/01942638.2015.1101043

Graham, F., Sinnott, K. A., Snell, D. L., Martin, R., & Freeman, C. (2013). A more "normal" life: Residents', family, staff, and managers' experience of active support at a residential facility for people with physical and intellectual impairments. *Journal of Intellectual and Developmental Disability*, *38*(3), 256–264. https://doi.org/10.3109/13668250.2013.805738

Graham, F., Williman, J., Jones, B., Ingham, T., Snell, D., Ranta, A., & Ziviani, J. (2019). *Coaching caregivers of children with developmental disability: A cluster RCT (19/617)* [Research Grant]. New Zealand: Health Research Council.

Grant, A. M., & Gerrard, B. (2019). Comparing problem-focused, solution-focused and combined problem-focused/solution-focused coaching approach: Solution-focused coaching questions mitigate the negative impact of dysfunctional attitudes. *Coaching: An International Journal of Theory, Research and Practice*, 1–17. https://doi.org/10.1080/17521882.2019.1599030

Greber, C., Ziviani, J., & Rodger, S. (2007). The Four Quadrant Model of facilitated learning (Part 1): Using teaching-learning approaches in occupational therapy. *Australian Occupational Therapy Journal*, *54*(Suppl. 1), 1–9. https://doi.org/10.1111/j.1440-1630.2007.00662.x

Greenberg, G., Ganshorn, K., & Danilkewich, A. (2001). Solution-focused therapy: Counseling model for busy family physicians. *Canadian Family Physician*, *47*(11), 2289. Retrieved from www.cfp.ca/content/47/11/2289.abstract.

Gzil, F., Lefeve, C., Cammelli, M., Pachoud, B., Ravaud, J. F., & Leplege, A. (2007). Why is rehabilitation not yet fully person-centred and should it be more person-centred? *Disability and Rehabilitation*, *29*(20–21), 1616–1624. https://doi.org/10.1080/09638280701618620

Imms, C., Adair, B., Keen, D., Ullenhag, A., Rosenbaum, P., & Granlund, M. (2016). "Participation": A systematic review of language, definitions, and constructs used in intervention research with children with disabilities. *Developmental Medicine & Child Neurology*, *58*(1), 29–38. https://doi.org/10.1111/dmcn.12932

Imms, C., Granlund, M., Wilson, P., Steenbergen, B., Rosenbaum, P., & Gordon, A. (2017). Participation, both a means and an end: A conceptual analysis of processes and outcomes in childhood disability. *Developmental Medicine & Child Neurology, 59*(1), 16–25. https://doi.org/10.1111/dmcn.13237

Jones, E., Perry, J., Lowe, K., Allen, D., Toogood, S., & Felce, D. (1996). *Active support: A handbook for planning daily activities and support arrangements for people with learning disabilities.* Cardiff: Welsh Centre for Learning Disabilities and Applied Research Unit.

Kessler, D., Walker, I., Sauve-Schenk, K., & Egan, M. (2019). Goal setting dynamics that facilitate or impede a client-centered approach. *Scandinavian Journal of Occupational Therapy, 26*(5), 315–324. https://doi.org/10.1080/11038128.2018.1465119

King, G., Servais, M., Shepherd, T. A., Willoughby, C., Bolack, L., Moodie, S., . . . McNaughton, N. (2017). A listening skill educational intervention for pediatric rehabilitation clinicians: A mixed-methods pilot study. *Developmental Neurorehabilitation, 20*(1), 40–52. https://doi.org/10.3109/17518423.2015.1063731

Kiresuk, T. J., & Sherman, R. E. (1968). Goal attainment scaling: A general method for evaluating comprehensive community mental health programs. *Community Mental Health Journal, 4*(6), 443–453. https://doi.org/10.1007/BF01530764

Kolehmainen, N., MacLennan, G., Ternent, L., Duncan, E., Duncan, E., Ryan, S., . . . Francis, J. (2012). Using shared goal setting to improve access and equity: A mixed methods study of the Good Goals intervention in children's occupational therapy. *Implementation Science, 7*(1), 76. https://doi.org/10.1186/1748-5908-7-76

Kolehmainen, N., Marshall, J., Hislop, J., Fayed, N., Kay, D., Ternent, L., & Pennington, L. (2019). Implementing participation-focused services: A study to develop the Method for using Audit and Feedback in Participation Implementation (MAPi). *Child: Care, Health and Development, 16*, 37–45. https://doi.org/10.1111/cch.12723

Law, M., Baptiste, S., Carswell, A., McColl, A., Polatajko, H., & Pollock, N. (2005). *COPM: Canadian occupational performance measure* (4th ed.). Ottawa, ON: CAOT Publications ACE.

Law, M., & Barker-Dunbar, S. (2007). Person-environment-occupation model. In S. Barker-Dunbar (Ed.), *Occupational therapy models for intervention with children and families.* Thorofare, NJ: Slack.

Law, M., Cooper, B., Strong, B., Stewart, D., Rigby, P., & Letts, L. (1996). The Person-Environment Occupation model: A transactive approach to occupational performance. *Canadian Journal of Occupational Therapy, 63*(1), 9–23. https://doi.org/10.1177/000841749606300103

Levack, W., Dean, S., Mcpherson, K., & Siegert, R. (2006a). How clinicians talk about the application of goal planning to rehabilitation for people with brain injury: Variable interpretations of value and purpose. *Brain Injury, 20*(13–14), 1439–1449. https://doi.org/10.1080/02699050601118422

Levack, W., Dean, S., Siegert, R., & Mcpherson, K. (2006b). Purposes and mechanisms of goal planning in rehabilitation: The need for a critical distinction. *Disability and Rehabilitation, 28*(12), 741–749. https://doi.org/10.1080/09638280500265961

Levack, W., Taylor, K., Siegert, R., Dean, S., McPherson, K., & Weatherall, M. (2006). Is goal planning in rehabilitation effective? A systematic review. *Clinical Rehabilitation, 20*, 739–755. https://doi.org/10.1177/0269215506070791

Litchfield, R., & MacDougall, C. (2002). Professional issues for physiotherapists in family-centred and community-based settings. *Australian Journal of Physiotherapy, 48*, 105–112. https://doi.org/10.1016/s0004-9514(14)60204-x

Locke, E., & Latham, G. P. (1984). *Goal setting: A motivational technique that works*. Englewood Cliffs, NJ: Prentice-Hall.

McDougall, J., & Wright, V. (2009). The ICF-CY and Goal Attainment Scaling: Benefits of their combined use for pediatric practice. *Disability & Rehabilitation, 31*(16), 1362–1372. https://doi.org/10.1080/09638280802572973

McPherson, K. M., Kayes, N. M., & Kersten, P. (2014). MEANING as a smarter approach to goals in rehabilitation. In R. Siegert & W. Levack (Eds.), *Rehabilitation goal setting: Theory, practice and evidence* (pp. 105–119). London: CRC Press.

Mezirow, J., & Taylor, E. (Eds.). (2009). *Transformative learning in practice: Insights from community, workplace and higher education*. San Francisco, CA: Jossey-Bass.

Michie, S., van Stralen, M. M., & West, R. (2011). The behaviour change wheel: A new method for characterising and designing behaviour change interventions. *Implementation Science, 6*(1), 42. https://doi.org/10.1186/1748-5908-6-42

Murray, A., Hall, A., Williams, G. C., McDonough, S. M., Ntoumanis, N., Taylor, I., . . . Matthews, J. (2019). Assessing physiotherapists' communication skills for promoting patient autonomy for self-management: Reliability and validity of the communication evaluation in rehabilitation tool. *Disability and Rehabilitation, 41*(14), 1699–1705. https://doi.org/10.1080/09638288.2018.1443159

Novak, I., Morgan, C., McNamara, L., & Te Velde, A. (2019). Best practice guidelines for communicating to parents the diagnosis of disability. *Early Human Development, 139*, 104841. https://doi.org/10.1016/j.earlhumdev.2019.104841

Ogourtsova, T., O'Donnell, M., De Souza Silva, W., & Majnemer, A. (2019). Health coaching for parents of children with developmental disabilities: A systematic review. *Developmental Medicine & Child Neurology, 61*, 1259–1265. https://doi.org/10.1111/dmcn.14206

Oxford University Press. (2019). *Lexico dictionary*. Retrieved from www.lexico.com/en/definition/sympathy

Randall, K. E., & McEwen, I. R. (2000). Writing patient-centered functional goals. *Physical Therapy, 80*(12), 1197–1203. https://doi.org/10.1093/ptj/80.12.1197

reflection. (n.d.). *Merriam-Webster.com*. Retrieved January 14, 2020 from www.merriam-webster.com/dictionary/reflection

Rosenbaum, P., & Gorter, J. (2012). The "F-words" in childhood disability: I swear this is how we should think! *Child: Care, Health and Development, 38*(4), 457–463. https://doi.org/10.1111/j.1365-2214.2011.01338.x

Rutherford Turnbull III, H., Beegle, G., & Stowe, M. J. (2001). The core concepts of disability policy affecting families who have children with disabilities. *Journal of Disability Policy Studies, 12*(3), 133–143. https://doi.org/10.1177/104420730101200302

Shapiro, S., & Carlson, L. (2017). What is mindfulness? In S. Shapiro & L. Carlson (Eds.), *The art and science of mindfulness: Integrating mindfulness into psychology and the helping professions* (2nd ed., pp. 9–20). Washington, DC: American Psychological Association.

Steenbeek, D., Ketelaar, M., Lindeman, E., Galama, K., & Gorter, J. W. (2010). Interrater reliability of Goal Attainment Scaling in rehabilitation of children with cerebral palsy. *Archives of Physical Medicine & Rehabilitation, 91*(3), 429–435. https://doi.org/10.1016/j.apmr.2009.10.013

Taylor, R. (2008). *The intentional relationship: Occupational therapy and use of self*. Philadel-
phia, PA: FA Davis.
Tennant, A. (2007). Goal Attainment Scaling: Current methodological challenges. *Disability and
Rehabilitation, 29*(20–21), 1–6. https://doi.org/10.1080/09638280701618828
World Health Organization. (2001). *International Classification of Functioning, Disability and
Health (ICF)*. Geneva: World Health Organization.

Chapter 4
Fidelity processes

Fiona Graham and Jenny Ziviani

Fidelity, in the context of health interventions, refers to the extent to which an intervention is implemented as intended (Hoffmann et al., 2014). As such, fidelity allows us to understand and monitor the delivery of interventions. It also allows researchers to be confident about what intervention was delivered when making claims about the validity of research findings on effectiveness (Graham, Ziviani, Kennedy-Behr, Kessler, & Hui, 2018).

Rehabilitation practitioners are highly attuned to the importance of individualising care, according to client needs, preferences, and contexts, to achieve person-centred outcomes. The value we confer to individualised care, however, can make the idea of standardising interventions feel uncomfortable. While acknowledging this practice reality, it is, nevertheless, important to determine if an intervention was implemented as intended in order to understand clearly if the intervention actually works, for whom, and under what conditions.

Knowledge of specific intervention components and standards of delivery are necessary for empirical analysis of interventions. This is an essential element of evidence-based practice (Mowbray, 2003) and includes also clarifying what we should not do in relation to specific interventions (Novak & Honan, 2019). Fidelity 'processes' comprise a broad range of strategies embedded in study design and/ or service delivery protocols that assist in monitoring and enhancing fidelity to interventions. Fidelity processes may include the extent of practitioner training in an intervention and the review of implementation of intervention sessions against fidelity measures or systems to elevate practitioner skills when low intervention fidelity is identified.

We know that practitioners seldom apply single interventions in isolation and instead draw from an eclectic mix of knowledge when engaging with individual clients (Bond, Evans, Salyers, Williams, & Kim, 2000). This makes sense in clinical practice given the wide range of client, practitioner, and contextual circumstances that exist. Yet, when we know the extent to which an intervention was implemented in its pure form (i.e., with fidelity), we can make sense of positive versus negative research findings and clinical outcomes. We can begin to understand if poor treatment results with clients are due to incorrect application of the intervention or a failure of the intervention to achieve the intended outcome for a particular client or population (Jelsma, Mertens, Forsberg, & Forsberg, 2015). By considering the outcomes we observe with a client, how the client responded to the intervention, and what we as practitioners did (including how well and how often we did it), we are able to refine interventions, improve on training, and clarify the populations for whom and contexts in which interventions such as OPC are most useful (Bond et al., 2000). As practitioners, we should also examine our specific intervention behaviours and reflect on what we do, don't do, or would like to do better with particular clients. The OPC fidelity processes and measures described in this chapter provide guidance for this reflection and learning process. These are described for independent researchers of OPC alongside practical strategies for practitioners seeking to evaluate their application of OPC. Minimum training criteria is described, with links to online training materials (beyond this book) provided. Fidelity information is summarised in the Template for Intervention Description and Replication (TIDieR; Hoffman et al., 2014) in Appendix E.

KEY MESSAGES

- Fidelity is important for understanding if OPC has been implemented as intended and if clients have responded to it as intended.
- The OPC Fidelity Measure is a key tool in establishing if OPC has been applied as intended, in both clinical and research settings. It enables us to reflect on our use of OPC and to understand which aspects of OPC work well, for which clients and in which contexts.

REFLECTIVE QUESTIONS

- How will you know when you are enacting OPC as it was intended? You may find it helpful to note down your answers to these questions before you begin reading.
- If you are a researcher, why is an understanding of fidelity processes pertinent to OPC important? If you are a practitioner, how will your understanding of OPC fidelity influence your practice?

A FIDELITY FRAMEWORK

Fidelity processes outlined in this chapter are organised according to the framework proposed by the Treatment Fidelity Workgroup of the National Institute of Health's Behaviour Change Consortium (Bellg et al., 2004). Within this framework study design (when engaging in research), training providers, delivery of intervention, and client enactment are identified. In this chapter, issues relevant to each of these strategies, with the exception of study design, will be addressed. Study design is dependent on the nature of the research questions being posed and hence outside the scope of this book.

Practitioners bring a wide range of skills and life experiences to their work, including to the learning of OPC, which may only partially reflect their formal qualifications. With this diversity among practitioners in mind, we focus on bodies of knowledge rather than professional qualifications in describing the background training for implementing OPC.

WHAT PRACTITIONER BACKGROUND TRAINING IS NEEDED?

In Chapter 2 of this manual, the core theories underpinning OPC, and therefore relevant to practitioners' application of OPC, are described briefly. The introduction to each body of knowledge in that chapter is intended as a starting point in preparation for learning OPC. Some practitioners will be well versed in these theories and models, while others will need to extend their reading beyond Chapter 2 to gain a more complete understanding of the concepts. In Chapter 5, key threshold concepts are distilled from these models and applied using case examples and video demonstrations (available online). The material in both Chapters 2 and 5 may be helpful to readers as a way of examining the fullness of their prerequisite understanding and knowledge for OPC. In the next section, we outline how to access further training in OPC, beyond material provided here.

Along with familiarisation and training in OPC, practitioners may also find that training in cognate approaches such as Motivational Interviewing (MI: Miller & Rollnick, 2002), Solution-Focused Therapy (SFT: de Shazer, 1984), or Acceptance Commitment Therapy (ACT: Hayes, Strosahl, & Kelly, 2012) and generic coaching skills will refine their skills in the use of autonomy-supportive communications with clients. Occupational performance analysis skills may be enhanced through training in interventions in which this is a core strategy, such as the Perceive Recall Plan Perform System of Task Analysis (Chapparo & Ranka, 2007) and the Cognitive

Orientation to Daily Occupational Performance (CO-OP: Missiuna, Mandich, Polatajko, & Malloy-Miller, 2001).

Knowledge about the health conditions specific to the client group with which practitioners are working is needed when employing OPC because professional expertise can inform the direction of performance analysis and how information can best be shared with clients. The primary expertise of the practitioner in OPC, however, is in coaching skills within rehabilitation contexts: engaging with clients to support their goal achievement, decision-making, and action toward occupational and participatory goals. Traditional bodies of knowledge such as mind and body systems, health condition specific knowledge, task analysis, and learning processes remain important background knowledge. This knowledge can be drawn upon to assist practitioners' questioning but is seldom explicitly 'taught' to clients in OPC. Instead, the emphasis is on eliciting client knowledge, insights, and ability to access information. In situations when practitioner knowledge (e.g., about health conditions) is imparted, specific strategies are used to minimise practitioner authority and maintain client expertise and agency, including seeking out additional information (see Chapter 3 for a detailed explanation of how traditional professional knowledge is applied within OPC).

ARE THERE PREREQUISITE PRACTITIONER COMPETENCIES FOR OPC?

Some practitioners appear more suited to OPC than others. Pre-professional students and novice as well as experienced practitioners have all been observed applying OPC skilfully, suggesting that age and years of experience are not necessarily key practitioner variables. Instead, practitioners who are rapid adopters of OPC appear to be those who have already integrated (or are 'ready, willing, and able' to do so) the threshold concepts of OPC described in Chapter 5.

HOW IS OPC TRAINING DELIVERED?

Training in OPC is currently available in a range of formats, lengths, and levels of difficulty depending on the purposes of training and experience of trainees. Here we outline how OPC training is delivered for each purpose, including strategies to minimise implementation drift.

Practitioner training

Practitioners may become trained in OPC through participating in workshops, undertaking an online course, or pursuing independent study of published materials. OPC workshops are standardised, ranging in length and complexity from one to five days. Workshops are taught by members of the OPC Trainers' Network listed on the official OPC website (www.otago.ac.nz/opc/training). OPC Trainers' Network membership is clearly stated on all training advertising and material. Training in these workshops includes didactic teaching using standardised materials, in vivo demonstration by trainers, video examples of OPC, small group casework, role play with in vivo coaching of training attendees, and self- and peer-assessment of fidelity. Workshops are delivered in-person, via videoconference, or with a mix of in-person and videoconference formats. Online, asynchronous coursework for OPC training is currently under development and will be publicly available from mid-2020 (see www.otago.ac.nz/opc).

Completion of any of these training options does not confer competency in OPC. While certificates of attendance at training may be issued, these do not attest to skill development in OPC. The reflective practitioner continually self-evaluates and reflects on their practice using OPC. Fidelity to OPC is assured only through evaluation of OPC fidelity using the OPC Fidelity Measure (OPC-FM), which is described in detail in this chapter and available in Appendix A. The OPC-FM is designed for self-assessment or external observer use. For research examining the effectiveness of OPC, OPC-FM raters should have completed training to train-the-trainer level (listed as members of the OPC Trainers' Network; www.otago.ac.nz/opc/training). OPC trainers may be available for online text-based support or individual training in OPC at their discretion.

Researcher training

For research purposes, we currently recommend training to be at least 24 hours in length, with a combination of self-study, in-person training, videoconference follow-up in small groups, and self- and peer evaluation of fidelity with individual feedback from peers and members of the OPC Trainers' Network. Training is ideally spaced over several weeks, with application with clients between training sessions. Fidelity above a minimum of 80% total score on the OPC-FM is recommended prior to study commencement.

Minimising implementation drift

Regular peer review of live or recorded sessions and self- or peer-rated OPC-FM are recommended to ensure OPC fidelity in service delivery contexts and research studies. Drift and contamination of interventions are common in both clinical and research situations for the application of a single intervention (Hall, Staiger,

Simpson, Best, & Lubman, 2016). Researchers and practitioners should consider implementing procedures to monitor with systems in place to top-up training, especially if fidelity falls below 80% on the OPC-FM. Strategies to support the fidelity with which OPC is delivered in clinical settings or pragmatic trials are described in this chapter in relation to monitoring fidelity and in Chapter 6 in relation to knowledge translation strategies.

Tailoring of training

To date, OPC training has not been formally tailored to specific professions or level of professional training. For reasons already described, the emphasis of OPC training is on evaluation of competence (by using the OPC-FM) rather than standardised 'dosage' of training for specific professional groups. Studies are currently underway to evaluate the effectiveness of OPC training via online and in-person training formats in establishing OPC competency for clinical and pre-professional populations (Chien & Graham, 2018; Graham et al., 2019).

Training of trainers in OPC

The following guidelines on training requirements for OPC are provided as a means of ensuring that what is proposed as OPC conforms to what has been developed and presented in this book. Members of the OPC Trainers' Network have undertaken at least 40 hours training in OPC and instruction in teaching of OPC, provided video evidence of consistently high fidelity (>80% on the OPC-FM), and demonstrated an understanding of underlying theories. Members commit to biennial training, including fidellty review assessment (to monitor trainer skills), to remain endorsed as OPC trainers on the OPC website (www.otago.ac.nz/opc) and contribute to the ongoing development of OPC resources. A cost-recovery fee is charged to all trainers for use of OPC standardised training material, with the exception of research-related training. Fees are paid directly to the University of Otago for the maintenance and development of OPC resources, research and dissemination.

WHAT DOSAGE OF OPC IS REQUIRED TO EFFECT CHANGE?

Dosage, sometimes referred to as exposure, measures how much of the intervention was delivered. Of particular interest is the minimal dosage required in order to elicit a level of client response that will lead to the desired outcomes of an intervention. The optimal 'dosage' of OPC (session number and length of session) is yet to be determined but is likely to vary for health populations, service delivery contexts, and individual clients. The number of sessions reported to date are four (Bernie, Graham, May, & Williams, 2019, May; Hui, Snider, & Couture, 2016; Kennedy-Behr, Rodger, Graham, & Mickan, 2013), six, eight (Graham, Rodger, & Ziviani, 2013a), ten (Graham, Rodger, & Ziviani, 2010), and twelve (Graham et al., 2010). One study increased session numbers from eight to ten in response to client request (Kessler, Ineza, Patel, Phillips, & Dubouloz, 2014). Another series of studies decreased the maximal session number from twelve (Graham et al., 2010) to ten (Graham et al., 2013a) based on clinical impressions of maximal effect in an earlier study. Sessions continue until goal/s are achieved to the satisfaction of the client, with no subsequent goals arising.

The interval between sessions has most commonly been a week, with tapering after initial sessions to fortnightly/monthly, at clients' request. It appears that the in-depth reflection, observation, and behaviour change stimulated in clients by OPC often requires practice time of more than one week before benefiting from further coaching.

WHAT DELIVERY FORMATS ARE SUITABLE FOR OPC?

Occupational Performance Coaching has so far been delivered in person 1:1 and via telehealth (telephone and/or videoconference)(Graham et al., 2010; Kessler, Dawson, & Anderson, 2018; Nott, Wiseman, Pike, & Seymour, 2019). Advantages and disadvantages were identified for telephone versus videoconference formats. Although telephone delivery lacked visual feedback, it had uninterrupted and real-time audio, enabling more natural flow to coaching conversations. For both telephone and videoconference delivery, performance analysis becomes more client-led as practitioners become almost entirely dependent on descriptions of situations provided by clients (see Chapter 7 for clinical stories on the use of OPC via tele-technologies).

Conceptually OPC could also be used with groups of clients, given it is already used with more than one client present with a direct common interest (see Chapter 3 where application of OPC with multiple clients is discussed). The adult learning basis of OPC (see Chapter 2), in which facilitated reflection and self-discovery are key tenets, lends itself to group delivery formats where there is some commonality to group members goals, challenges, and learner needs (Alrø & Dahl, 2015). Group delivery of any form of coaching is more complex than 1:1 delivery hence some tailoring of OPC, such as initial group contract and explicit session structure, may be needed.

HOW IS FIDELITY TO OPC MEASURED?

Three tools guide OPC intervention fidelity: The OPC Fidelity Measure (see Appendix A), the OPC Session Schedule (see Appendix F), and the OPC Casenote Audit Tool (see Appendix G). The OPC-FM is the formal measure of fidelity, covering all key practitioner and client behaviours expected during OPC. Research studies investigating the effects and effectiveness of OPC are expected to report OPC-FM scores alongside study findings. The OPC Session Schedule and OPC Casenote Audit Tool are primarily intended as tools to assist practitioners' implementation of OPC. The OPC Session Schedule indicates session-by-session expectations of OPC-related practitioner behaviours. The OPC Casenote Audit Tool provides a checklist of expected documentation following OPC sessions, with the intention of guiding practitioner behaviour and as a resource for casenote audit as a means of establishing proxy fidelity when session observation or recording is not possible.

OPC Fidelity Measure

The OPC-FM (see Appendix A) is designed to measure the extent to which OPC is implemented as intended. It has been developed and tested using recommended methods (Mowbray, 2003), resulting in several (unpublished) iterations of the tool. An explicit design intention in creating the OPC-FM has been brevity and simplicity, given the challenges that ensue when observational measures become too onerous and detailed (e.g., non-use) (Caperton, Atkins, & Imel, 2018).

The OPC-FM has 18 items, of which 14 focus on practitioner behaviour and four on client behaviour (response). Three items are only applicable to sessions subsequent to an initial session, as they relate to enactment of client behaviours discussed in earlier sessions. Therefore, the total possible raw score differs for initial and subsequent sessions.

Each item of the OPC-FM is rated on a four-point scale indicating both occurrence of practitioner or client behaviours and quality of behaviour. Detailed item and scale descriptions are provided as part of the measure. A score of zero indicates non-occurrence of practitioner and client behaviours and a score of one to three indicates the quality with which behaviour has occurred.

Quality of practitioner and client behaviour is rated as one (low), two (moderate), or three (high). Throughout testing (Gadkari, Graham, & Mulcahey, 2018, Graham, Rodger, & Ziviani, 2013b), the wording of items was refined and items condensed. Detailed descriptions and examples of each level of rating are provided in the

OPC-FM Item Descriptors (see Appendix A). Briefly, for each item, a score of one indicates that there was poor use of a behaviour to the extent that it is very unlikely that a therapeutic effect toward goal achievement will occur. A score of two indicates that moderate evidence of the behaviour was observed, however some opportunities to extend the use of the item behaviour were missed, to the extent that goal progress is likely to be limited. A score of three indicates that almost all opportunities to apply the item were taken and fully utilised, to the extent that they are likely to substantially impact sustainable, goal-related actions and, thus, substantially influence goal achievement.

Three distinguishing items (15–18) are included in the OPC-FM to differentiate OPC from other interventions (for example, Item 15, 'Therapist provides advice without implicit or stated permission'). Component differentiation provides demarcation between the particular elements of the intervention and elements that may be present in other approaches. These items explicitly indicate practitioner behaviours that are at odds with OPC, thus reflect what a practitioner using OPC should *not* do. High scores in these items reflect low-quality implementation of OPC. It is possible that a practitioner executes other OPC behaviours well *and* also engages in distinguishing behaviour items (see Appendix A). The effect on fidelity scores in this case would be a lower overall fidelity score than if distinguishing items were not part of the measure. Distinguishing item scores are reversed when summating scores.

Client response items are also included in the OPC-FM in recognition of the influence of client response on adherence and intervention outcomes (Carroll et al., 2007). Client response (also termed participant involvement) assesses the extent that participants are actively engaged in the intervention process (Carroll et al., 2007). Client response to practitioner behaviours when implementing an intervention are integral to fidelity, given that client response (reception of practitioner behaviour and subsequent enactment of change) is a critical part of the mechanism of impact (Moore et al., 2015). Client response can also be thought of as a moderator of the effect of an intervention (Carroll et al., 2007). Highly skilled practitioners in a rehabilitation intervention such as OPC modify their application of techniques in response to judgements of client needs (e.g., clients' readiness for change, literacy level) in order to achieve the same effect (Moore et al., 2015). In the case of OPC the effect being sought is goal progress.

Inclusion of client response items in the OPC-FM (Items 11 to 14) should be examined in relation to practitioner adherence (Bond et al., 2000) in order to distinguish between practitioner implementation and client enactment. For researchers, clarification of client response assists in the interpretation of findings, including determining if practitioner behaviours in OPC elicit the intended client response with specific populations and in specific contexts. For practitioners using the OPC-FM as a self- or peer assessment, consideration of the relationship between practitioner behaviours and client responses can be a valuable source of feedback on the extent of use of practitioner behaviours.

How have client perspectives of fidelity been gathered?

The client experience of engaging in OPC and how this translates to enactment of responses to OPC outside of therapy sessions is also an important fidelity consideration (Bellg et al., 2004). To date, parents' perspectives of OPC have been garnered using surveys (Graham, Rodger, Ziviani, & Jones, 2016) and semi-structured interviews (see Chapter 6 for further details). Features of OPC that parents identified as influencing their behaviours, and subsequently leading to goal progress, were the meaningfulness of goals, the degree of personal reflection and thinking required, along with a sense of supportive accountability to act. The extent to which these experiences apply to other recipients of OPC requires further research (Kessler, Walker, Sauve-Schenk, & Egan, 2019).

HOW IS OPC FIDELITY MONITORED?

Monitoring of intervention fidelity over time, within research studies or clinical programme implementation, is a critical aspect of ensuring fidelity is maintained. The OPC-FM has been designed with clinical and research applications in mind, with attention to brevity and the potential for use as a self- or peer assessment.

External observer monitoring

Observation of video footage by external raters is considered the gold standard in assessing fidelity, as this allows for the capture of what actually occurs in an intervention encounter (Proctor et al., 2011). Ideally OPC fidelity for research purposes is evaluated from video recordings of all intervention sessions by an external observer with advanced training in OPC. Our experience in use of the OPC-FM suggests that video recordings are ideal as they show non-verbal responses as well as verbal interactions. Recording all sessions minimises the potential for differences (unintended bias) in the application of OPC in recorded versus unrecorded sessions. All recordings can then be rated or randomly selected for rating.

The expectation of recording of OPC sessions can become a significant barrier to recruitment in research trials in our experience, particularly in the current digital environment. Clients or practitioners may have concerns about protection of privacy despite assurance of best practice data security. Audio recordings may be a more acceptable form of recording. Further research is required to determine the agreement of OPC-FM ratings between audio only versus audio plus video recordings.

Self-monitoring of fidelity

If recording of OPC sessions is not possible, it is suggested that the OPC-FM be used as a self-report tool by the intervention practitioner. Self-monitoring is a practical and economical approach to the maintenance of fidelity and a means of minimising intervention drift over time (Fox & Riconscente, 2008). Self-monitoring can be a useful prompt for feedback and reflection on adherence to OPC (Gadkari et al., 2018). The self-regulation process acts as a mechanism to form the habit of high fidelity of implementation, which maintains behaviours over time (Fox & Riconscente, 2008). On this theoretical premise, the OPC-FM is proposed as a way for practitioners to self-monitor fidelity to OPC and embed fidelity monitoring into routine quality assurance processes such as supervision, clinical audit-feedback cycles, and in-house training. However, in lieu of research on the agreement between self-report and external observer ratings using the OPC-FM, for research purposes external observer rating is recommended whenever possible. Both practitioner self-report and observation of delivery can inform fidelity, however relying on self-report alone can be misleading (Brosan, Reynolds, & Moore, 2008).

Ensuring fidelity in either clinical or research environments requires multiple strategies, embedded in training and intervention delivery processes and maintained over time. Underpinning the success of these strategies, however, is the reflective practitioner, seeking with curiosity to examine their practices and adopt different ways of working based on feedback and insight. In this chapter we have presented those strategies used with success in research to date and recommended in the literature. Chapter 7 extends on some of the fidelity material in describing how OPC has been applied by a range of services, including embedding OPC training and monitoring processes as part of 'usual care'.

HOW CAN OPC BE TAILORED?

Tailoring (or adaptation) refers to modifications of an intervention to accommodate the needs of specific health populations or service delivery contexts, but with fidelity to the underlying principles of an intervention (Moore et al., 2008). Tailoring of an intervention is an important step in the development of innovations which can ultimately enhance an intervention, but it can be confused with low fidelity or a misunderstanding of an intervention's principles or application; hence, the importance of adherence to the training guidelines prior to evaluation of OPC in clinical or research contexts. We propose key questions which should be considered in determining if a modification to the OPC intervention procedures described in this book might be appropriate, including:

- Are these adaptations consistent with the theories underpinning OPC (in Chapter 2)?
- Are these adaptations consistent with the mechanisms of impact of OPC, particularly practitioner resource, as outlined in the logic model (Chapter 4)?
- Do these adaptations encourage high-quality OPC practitioner and client behaviours?
- Do these adaptations avoid requiring the practitioner to enact any of the *distinguishing* ('don't do') behaviours as outlined in the OPC-FM (Appendix A)?

If the answer is 'no' to any of these questions, then the adaptation of OPC moves beyond tailoring to become a new and different intervention. Components of the new intervention might most appropriately be described as 'informed by' aspects of OPC, with recognition that the new intervention will develop and require an independent evidence base. Next we address common questions about how OPC is currently applied (with different emphases for different populations) and delineate what is considered standard OPC, what might be described as tailoring of OPC, and what might be considered to have become a different intervention.

Are outcome measures considered an adaptation to OPC?

Formal measures of occupational performance and participation are best practice clinically and in research. While not inherent to OPC intervention, formal outcome measures are recommended. Research on OPC to date has used the Canadian Occupational Performance Measure (COPM: Law et al., 1990) or Goal Attainment Scaling (GAS: Kiresuk & Sherman, 1968) as individualised measures of goal progress (see Chapter 7 for more information). These measures continue to be recommended and are not considered a tailoring of OPC because they are not inherently a part of OPC.

Can I grade language and visual supports without tailoring OPC?

Adjustment of language complexity and the use of visual supports to guide the coaching process or share information is considered part of standard OPC. These communication strategies are viewed as a form of grading of OPC conversations to match a client's abilities. Central tenets of OPC of authentic relationships, an occupational/participatory focus, and client-led reflection, analysis, and decision-making remain unchanged by the use of these strategies. This kind of adjustment might be needed when clients have limited health (or general) literacy or have cognitive or communication impairments associated with their health conditions. For example, language can be simplified and cognitive demand reduced by offering clients two or three closed choices if they seem unable to process open-ended questions. A question such as *"What might help in this situation?"* can be less abstract by phrasing it as *"How can you change the way you do this task?"* When using more narrowly funnelled questions in this way, it is important to be aware that this may not be the direction the client is considering and to change the direction of questioning accordingly.

Similarly, more complex language might be used with clients with specialised skills (such as health or education professionals) or those with advanced literacy. Visual supports (graphics, diagrams) can be helpful for many clients when discussing abstract or novel concepts. Frequently reported visual supports include visuals showing OPC processes and principles (for example see OPC Process, Appendix B) or graphics specific to particular health conditions or other explanatory factors related to goal achievement and arising from coaching conversations. For example, a practitioner working with families of children with autism spectrum disorder using OPC may arrive at a point during coaching where parents develop insight as to the impact of children's arousal level on successful participation in home life. With parents' permission, sharing a graphic illustrating how arousal level fluctuates might augment parents' reflection and insight into ways in which children can be successfully supported to self-regulate during daily routines. Similarly, for adults post-stroke, the concept of neuroplasticity might be shared (with or without illustration) to help clients understand changes to their abilities and the value of re-engaging in life roles and activities. In both of these examples, interpretation and decision-making on application of knowledge is undertaken by clients. Thus clients, rather than practitioners, remain the agents of change. In contrast, prepared lists of activity or exercise suggestions, advice, or home programmes are at odds with the central tenets of OPC as, like direct instruction or training, these place agency with the practitioner rather than the client.

How is cultural diversity accommodated within OPC delivery?

Culturally specific activities, values, and perceptions can require tailoring of interventions in order to achieve the intended client outcomes. In a series of unpublished interviews for this book, reflections of early adopters of OPC who have been applying it with people of diverse cultures have been surprisingly consistent in the view that OPC needed little to no tailoring. Cultures with which OPC has been applied include Māori and Pakeha (non-Māori) New Zealanders, Aboriginal and non-Aboriginal Australians, French and English Canadians, Germans, Irish, Hong Kong Chinese, Taiwanese, Singaporeans, Italians, Iranians, and Israelis. Specific attention to relationships within OPC might be a key feature of OPC that supports this cross-cultural translation.

Tailoring of OPC for Māori is proposed to include the Hui process (Lacey, Huria, Beckert, Gilles, & Pitama, 2011), an overarching guide for culturally competent engagement with Māori. Like OPC, the Hui process emphasises relationship development but extends the making of connection (known as *whakawhanaungatanga*) to a reciprocal disclosure of personal information from the healthcare provider and client before the commencement of the main discussion. The Hui process is easily integrated into OPC for clients who identify as Māori and clearly aligns with the core tenets of OPC. It has been identified here as an example of cultural tailoring of OPC, rather than suggesting it works for all 'indigenous' cultures. In some cases, restrictive physical environments or human rights for people with disabilities in some societies may limit client response to OPC (Kahjoogh et al., 2019).

What therapeutic strategies are beyond tailoring of OPC?

In addition to the broad guidance on differentiating tailoring from low fidelity to OPC, special mention is made here of two types of adjustment that represent low fidelity – practitioner-led assessment prior to coaching and prescribed teaching or training within OPC. Both of these adaptations of OPC place agency with practitioners rather than clients, thus are inconsistent with the core principles of OPC. They emphasise practitioner bodies of knowledge as taking precedence and place the practitioner in control over the direction of therapy. They also imply an assumption that solutions to clients' achievement of their goals lies in these bodies of knowledge, be that the findings from practitioners' assessments or the training material.

While the sharing of information fits within OPC (see Chapter 3, Share domain), this is done in ways in which client agency is maintained and closely linked to clients' 'need to know'. Similarly, close analysis of one component of goal situations might warrant use of a formal assessment tool on rare occasions in OPC, however this would be embedded within a collaborative performance analysis (see Chapter 3,

Structure domain) in which the client is highly involved, has led the analysis up to that point, and given permission for the practitioner to explore an aspect of performance independently. Because performance is so innately wedded to context (and OPC goals are always context specific), it is difficult to conceive when a norm-referenced standardised assessment would add value to the identification of solutions within OPC. It is recognised, however, that there may be important reasons for norm-referenced standardised assessment in clinical practice outside of the application of OPC, such as diagnostic work-up, funding applications, or service entry criteria. An illustrative example of tailoring of OPC that is consistent with OPC principles that has recently been examined is the use of a brief version of OPC with parents waiting for diagnostic evaluation for autism spectrum disorder in Australia (Bernie et al., 2019).

CONCLUSION

This chapter details the fidelity processes for applying OPC in the way it was intended in both clinical and research contexts. Resources are provided to enable practitioners to assess, monitor, and report fidelity through video observation, self-assessment, and casenote auditing. Each of these tools is only as reliable as the user is informed about the theories, principles, and practices of OPC, also shared in this text. In addition, for research purposes, we currently recommend in-person training alongside independent study of OPC as provided here. The following chapter moves from the detailed process of fidelity to the threshold concepts which underpin the principles of OPC and are relevant in understanding what is common in its application in diverse situations.

REFERENCES

Alrø, H., & Dahl, P. N. (2015). Dialogic group coaching: Inspiration from transformative mediation. *Journal of Workplace Learning, 27*(7), 501–513. https://doi.org/10.1108/JWL-10-2014-0073

Bellg, A. J., Borrelli, B., Resnick, B., Hecht, J., Minicucci, D. S., Ory, M., . . . Czajkowski, S. (2004). Enhancing treatment fidelity in health behavior change studies: Best practices and recommendations from the NIH Behavior Change Consortium. *Health Psychology, 23*(5), 443–451.

Bernie, C., Graham, F., May, T., & Williams, K. (2019). *Feasibility of Occupational Performance Coaching for addressing child and family functional goals whilst waiting for Autism assessment in Melbourne Australia*. Paper presented at the 31st meeting of the European Academy of Childhood Disability, Paris, France.

Bond, G. R., Evans, L., Salyers, M. P., Williams, J., & Kim, H.-W. (2000). Measurement of fidelity in psychiatric rehabilitation. *Mental Health Services Research, 2*(2), 75–87. https://doi.org/10.1023/a:1010153020697

Brosan, L., Reynolds, S., & Moore, R. (2008). Self-evaluation of cognitive therapy performance: Do therapists know how competent they are? *Behavioural and Cognitive Psychotherapy, 36*(5), 581–587. https://doi.org/10.1017/S1352465808004438

Caperton, D. D., Atkins, D. C., & Imel, Z. E. (2018). Rating motivational interviewing fidelity from thin slices. *Psychology of Addictive Behaviors*, *32*(4), 434–441. https://doi.org/10.1037/adb0000359

Carroll, C., Patterson, M., Wood, S., Booth, S., Rick, J., & Balain, S. (2007). A conceptual framework for intervention fidelity. *Implementation Science*, *2*(40), 1–9. https://doi.org/10.1186/1748-5908-2-40

Chapparo, C., & Ranka, J. (2007). *The PRPP system: Intervention*. Lidcombe, AU: The University of Sydney.

Chien, C. W., & Graham, F. (2018). Limited evidence exists for the psychometric properties of child report measures that assess occupational performance in children ages 2–18 years. *Australian Occupational Therapy Journal*, *65*(5), 472–473. https://doi.org/10.1111/1440-1630.12531.

de Shazer, S. (1984). *Keys to solutions in brief therapy*. New York: Norton.

Fox, E., & Riconscente, M. (2008). Metacognition and self-regulation in James, Piaget, and Vygotsky. *Educational Psychology Review*, *20*(4), 373–389. https://doi.org/10.1007/s10648-008-9079-2

Gadkari, S., Graham, F., & Mulcahey, M. J. (2018). *Utility of the Occupational Performance Coaching fidelity measure (V2) as a self-assessment tool: A pilot study*. Paper presented at the American Occupational Therapy Conference, Salt Lake City, UT.

Graham, F., Rodger, S., & Ziviani, J. (2010). Enabling occupational performance of children through coaching parents: Three case reports. *Physical & Occupational Therapy in Pediatrics*, *30*(1), 4–15. https://doi.org/10.3109/01942630903337536

Graham, F., Rodger, S., & Ziviani, J. (2013a). Effectiveness of Occupational Performance Coaching in improving children's and mothers' performance and mothers' self-competence. *American Journal of Occupational Therapy*, *67*(1), 10–18. https://doi.org/10.5014/ajot.2013.004648

Graham, F., Rodger, S., & Ziviani, J. (2013b). *Occupational Performance Coaching: Determining intervention fidelity (02/13)* [Research Grant]. New Zealand: University of Otago Research Grant.

Graham, F., Rodger, S., Ziviani, J., & Jones, V. (2016). Strategies identified as effective by mothers during Occupational Performance Coaching. *Physical & Occupational Therapy in Pediatrics*, *36*(3), 247–259. https://doi.org/10.3109/01942638.2015.1101043

Graham, F., Williman, J., Jones, B., Ingham, T., Snell, D., Ranta, A., & Ziviani, J. (2019). *Coaching caregivers of children with developmental disability: A cluster RCT (19/617)* [Research Grant]. New Zealand: Health Research Council.

Graham, F., Ziviani, J., Kennedy-Behr, A., Kessler, D., & Hui, C. (2018). Fidelity of Occupational Performance Coaching: Importance of accuracy in intervention identification. *OTJR Occupation, Participation and Health*, *38*(1), 67–69. https://doi.org/10.1177/1539449217738926

Hall, K., Staiger, P. K., Simpson, A., Best, D., & Lubman, D. I. (2016). After 30 years of dissemination, have we achieved sustained practice change in motivational interviewing? *Addiction*, *111*(7), 1144–1150. https://doi.org/10.1111/add.13014

Hayes, S., Strosahl, K., & Kelly, W. (2012). *Acceptance and commitment therapy: The process and practice of mindful change* (2nd ed.). New York: Guilford Press.

Hoffmann, T. C., Glasziou, P. P., Boutron, I., Milne, R., Perera, R., Moher, D., . . . Johnston, M. (2014). Better reporting of interventions: Template for Intervention Description and Replication (TIDieR) checklist and guide. *British Medical Journal*, *348*, 1–12. https://doi.org/10.1136/bmj.g1687

Hui, C., Snider, L., & Couture, M. (2016). Self-regulation workshop and Occupational Performance Coaching with teachers: A pilot project. *Canadian Journal of Occupational Therapy*, *83*(2), 115–125. https://doi.org/10.1177/0008417415627665

Jelsma, J. G. M., Mertens, V. C., Forsberg, L., & Forsberg, L. (2015). How to measure motivational interviewing fidelity in randomized controlled trials: Practical recommendations. *Contemporary Clinical Trials*, *43*, 93–99. https://doi.org/10.1016/j.cct.2015.05.001

Kahjoogh, M., Kessler, D., Hosseini, S., Rassafiani, M., Akbarfahimi, N., Khankey, H., & Biglarian, A. (2019). Randomised controlled trial of Occupational Performance Coaching for mothers of children with cerebral palsy. *British Journal of Occupational Therapy*, *82*(4), 1–7. https://doi.org/10.1177/0308022618799944

Kennedy-Behr, A., Rodger, S., Graham, F., & Mickan, S. (2013). Creating enabling environments at preschool for children with developmental coordination disorder. *Journal of Occupational Therapy, Schools, & Early Intervention*, *6*(4), 301–313. https://doi.org/10.1080/19411243.2013.860760

Kessler, D., Dawson, D., & Anderson, N. (2018, October). *Is Occupational Performance Coaching for stroke survivors delivered via telerehabilitation (tele-OPC-stroke) feasible and acceptable to recipients?* Paper presented at the 11th World Stroke Congress, Montreal.

Kessler, D., Ineza, I., Patel, H., Phillips, M., & Dubouloz, C. (2014). Occupational Performance Coaching adapted for stroke survivors (OPC-Stroke): A feasibility evaluation. *Physical & Occupational Therapy in Geriatrics*, *32*(1), 42–57. https://doi.org/10.3109/02703181.2013.873845

Kessler, D., Walker, I., Sauve-Schenk, K., & Egan, M. (2019). Goal setting dynamics that facilitate or impede a client-centered approach. *Scandinavian Journal of Occupational Therapy*, *26*(5), 315–324. https://doi.org/10.1080/11038128.2018.1465119

Kiresuk, T. J., & Sherman, R. E. (1968). Goal Attainment Scaling: A general method for evaluating comprehensive community mental health programs. *Community Mental Health Journal*, *4*(6), 443–453. https://doi.org/10.1007/BF01530764

Lacey, C., Huria, T., Beckert, L., Gilles, M., & Pitama, S. (2011). The Hui Process: A framework to enhance the doctor-patient relationship with Maori. *The New Zealand Medical Journal (Online)*, *124*(1347).

Law, M., Baptiste, S., McColl, M., Opzoomer, A., Polatajko, H., & Pollock, N. (1990). The Canadian Occupational Performance Measure: An outcome measure for occupational therapy. *Canadian Journal of Occupational Therapy*, *57*(2), 82–87. https://doi.org/10.1177/000841749005700207

Miller, W., & Rollnick, S. (2002). *Motivational interviewing: Preparing people for change* (2nd ed.). New York: Guilford Press.

Missiuna, C., Mandich, A. D., Polatajko, H. J., & Malloy-Miller, T. (2001). Cognitive Orientation to Daily Occupational Performance (CO-OP): Part 1 – Theoretical foundations. *Physical & Occupational Therapy in Pediatrics*, *20*(2–3), 69–81. https://doi.org/10.1080/J006v20n02_05

Moore, G., Audrey, S., Barker, M., Bond, L., Bonell, C., Hardeman, W., . . . Baird, J. (2008). *Process evaluation of complex interventions: UK Medical Research Council (MRC) guidance*. Retrieved from https://mrc.ukri.org/documents/pdf/mrc-phsrn-process-evaluation-guidance-final/

Moore, G., Audrey, S., Barker, M., Bond, L., Bonell, C., Hardeman, W., . . . Baird, J. (2015). Process evaluation of complex interventions: Medical Research Council guidance. *British Medical Journal*, *350*, h1258. https://doi.org/10.1136/bmj.h1258

Mowbray, C. T. (2003). Fidelity criteria: Development, measurement, and validation. *The American Journal of Evaluation, 24*(3), 315–340. https://doi.org/10.1177/109821400302400303

Nott, M., Wiseman, L., Pike, S., & Seymour, T. (2019, July). *Stroke self-management supported by Occupational Therapy Coaching in rural New South Wales.* Paper presented at the Occupational Therapy Australia 28th National Conference and Exhibition: "Together Towards Tomorrow", Sydney, Australia.

Novak, I., & Honan, I. (2019). Effectiveness of paediatric occupational therapy for children with disabilities: A systematic review. *Australian Occupational Therapy Journal, 66*(3), 258–273. https://doi.org/10.1111/1440-1630.12573

Proctor, E., Silmere, H., Raghavan, R., Hovmand, P., Aarons, G., Bunger, A., . . . Hensley, M. (2011). Outcomes for implementation research: Conceptual distinctions, measurement challenges, and research agenda. *Administration and Policy in Mental Health and Mental Health Services Research, 38*(2), 65–76. https://doi.org/10.1007/s10488-010-0319-7

Chapter 5
Threshold concepts
Fiona Graham and Dorothy Kessler

Dr Dorothy Kessler, *currently an assistant professor in the School of Rehabilitation Therapy at Queen's University Canada, is an occupational therapist with over 30 years' experience working with older adults, primarily in the area of stroke rehabilitation. Dr Kessler tested OPC with people who have experienced stroke as part of her doctoral studies and is exploring its use with adults with other complex chronic conditions such as multiple sclerosis.*

Having described in detail the OPC format and procedures in Chapters 3 and 4, this chapter assists practitioners in developing their knowledge of key learning concepts that we believe students of OPC must grasp in order to apply it with effect. These learning concepts are described by some as 'threshold concepts' (Nicola-Richmond, Pépin, Larkin, & Taylor, 2018) – practices or understandings that are often troublesome, and sometimes counterintuitive, yet have the potential to be transformative aspects of knowledge, that once learnt are impossible to unlearn (Nicola-Richmond et al., 2018).

Through our observations of practitioners' and researchers' transitions to expert implementers of OPC, we have identified five threshold concepts for OPC. Once these five concepts have been grasped and a threshold effectively 'crossed', OPC practitioners are more likely to be able to integrate the information presented throughout this book. Learners who have crossed this metaphorical threshold of understanding may even experience a shift in their identity as practitioners or in how they define their professional roles. The five threshold learning concepts of OPC are:

1   High-trust partnerships are critical to coaching and are intentionally developed.

2   Meaningful goals are when dreams come true, rather than problems minimised.
3   Impairments rarely inform solutions. Enabling strategies can arise from anywhere.
4   Clients, rather than practitioners, are the agents of change in coaching.
5   Expertise in coaching lies in how we engage with people rather than what we know about them.

This chapter presents five cases formulated to illustrate each threshold concept in turn, highlighting the relevant insights, knowledge, and OPC skills which become accessible to the learner once this concept is understood. Links to online video footage of coaching examples (and transcripts of these) are provided in the eResources accompanying this book at www.routledge. com/9780367427962/eResource for each case for learners to watch/read and listen. All of these cases have been filmed with actors performing the role of clients and real occupational therapists in the role of a practitioner engaging in an OPC session.

For each concept, the reader is prompted to engage in reflection tasks to enhance self-awareness of their personal learning journey. Descriptions are provided of practitioners who have mastered each concept (these sections are titled concepts 'in action') to clarify the difference that knowing the concept makes on practice. Reflections from practitioners who recall their personal 'aha' moment as they crossed the learning threshold to gain these insights are also provided.

For learning purposes, we recommend that for each threshold concept, you follow the signposts which prompt you to:

- Commence by reading the illustrative case description and the brief explanation of the threshold concept prior to watching the online video (or reading the transcript thereof).

- Watch the video or read the transcript (see eResources).

- Complete reflection tasks as highlighted throughout each case and finish by reading practitioners' reflections about learning each of the threshold concepts.

KEY MESSAGES

- Implementing OPC requires practitioners to grasp a series of concepts related to engaging with clients and how we view our role. Once these concepts are understood, practitioners' competence in OPC and effectiveness with clients escalates.
- In some ways, the concepts presented here sit on a cusp between knowledge and insight. We can equip ourselves with the knowledge of OPC techniques and procedures, but gaining insight into the effect of these concepts on how we practise requires us to reflect on our current assumptions and ways of doing things.
- We believe that anyone can learn these concepts, but the timing in our professional lives needs to be right. Timing relates to our life experiences, temperament, professional training, and experiences.

REFLECTIVE PROMPTS

- As you read each of the following sections, reflect on how important you currently view the threshold concept to your practice. One way to do this is to ask yourself what other learner concepts are more and less important than the learner concepts presented here.
- Rate your agreement with each learning concept on a scale from one to ten. Try doing this before and again after reading each section and completing the learning activities. If you find your views have shifted, make notes on this shift in your thinking or discuss these ideas with colleagues.
- How would integration of these learning concepts impact on your work with clients?
- What specifically would be different in how you practise?

THRESHOLD CONCEPT #1: HIGH-TRUST PARTNERSHIPS ARE CRITICAL TO COACHING AND ARE INTENTIONALLY DEVELOPED

BOX 5.1   ILLUSTRATIVE CASE. MEET AROHA

Aroha has four children. The fourth child (Kahu) is six months old and was born prematurely with early signs of cerebral palsy – asymmetrical movement on one side of his body. Aroha lives in an extended family with strong expression of *tikanga* (Māori customs); the family speak a mix of Māori and English at home. There is a family culture of acceptance of everyone as they are, so Aroha is not concerned that Kahu is developing differently.

Kahu was born seven weeks early and was immediately admitted to the Special Care Baby Unit (SCBU) where he stayed for two weeks. Aroha disliked all the rules of the SCBU and is wary of health professionals. She has agreed to meet the occupational therapist once but suspects she is being checked up on.

As part of the SCBU follow-up services, Fiona, an occupational therapist, has been asked to monitor Kahu's development at home, initiate referrals as needed, and provide intervention to the child and family. Fiona is skilled in OPC but is also aware of her service's contractual obligations to monitor Kahu over the next three years.

What are high-trust partnerships?

Clients' trust of practitioners is essential if clients are to disclose what really matters to them and what gets in the way of achieving their goals. In the case of Aroha and Kahu, there is an active distrust of the practitioner to overcome from the outset. High-trust partnerships also accelerate the therapeutic process, leading to more rapid change for clients as the full picture of what is occurring is shared with the practitioner at earlier stages. Fiona is sitting with competing agendas, (1) to monitor Kahu's development *and* (2) to provide family-centred, developmentally supportive care, yet her success with both of these agendas rests on her ability to establish a high-trust partnership with Aroha at this first meeting. If this trust is to develop, Aroha will need to experience Fiona as being respectful of Aroha's strong sense of autonomy, relating her involvement with Aroha's family to what is most important to Aroha. Fiona will also need to convey that she is authentically invested in the wellbeing of Aroha's family.

 Watch how Fiona develops this trust with Aroha. Notice key points in the session when Fiona's comments appear to project trust *in* Aroha.

 Reflect on what you might have said that was either very different, or very similar, to Fiona's comments.

- What kinds of expression or wording might work well in your context?
- Write these statements or questions down to help make the wording accessible the next time you are focusing on partnership building when using OPC.

The power of high-trust partnerships

Once practitioners are able to develop high-trust partnerships with clients (including those whose lives and experiences are quite different to ours), they find that clients are much more engaged in the process of therapy. For Fiona and Aroha, this heightened engagement meant that Aroha allowed Fiona to see the family again. It also means that when it came to the developmentally related intervention with Kahu, Aroha was actively involved in figuring out how to encourage Kahu's movements rather than seeing this as 'the practitioners' job', an all too common dynamic.

Prioritising establishing a high-trust partnership does mean that therapy sometimes looks quite different to what a practitioner-directed therapy session would look like (this is what makes coaching such fun!). Enhancing client engagement isn't about sneaky ways to get clients to do what we want. It is about letting go of 'what we want' and being prepared to follow the clients' priorities. In 'usual care' (distinct from OPC), an early intervention session would start with a formal assessment of the child's function. This approach allows the practitioner to be comprehensive in her reporting of the child's impairments and may provide important baseline information for services, but it would do little to meet the needs of Aroha at this first visit. Had Fiona taken this approach, it is very likely that Aroha would refuse or fail to attend future appointments. Instead, Fiona centred her actions on what was important to Aroha and built on Aroha's observations of Kahu during nappy changing. She was then able to observe Kahu's motor skills as he participated in nappy changing with Aroha. Fiona was able to note that Kahu had a broad pattern of low muscle tone and reduced spontaneous movements in all limbs but especially in both legs. Aroha's observations that Kahu did not initiate any rolling movements during nappy changing and that he felt 'heavy' when being carried were astute. Both activities are excellent starting points for supporting Kahu's development and addressing Aroha's priorities, but undertaken in partnership with Aroha.

High-trust partnerships in action

 Think back to the video of Aroha and Fiona. How would you describe the qualities or style of Fiona's communication (e.g., wording, pace, tone)? What responses to this style of communication did you observe from Aroha? What would you like to explore in your own future relationship building with clients?

A key observation of practitioners who have prioritised relationship building in their practice is the distinctive way in which they listen mindfully to clients. These practitioners predominantly use open-ended questions and listen very attentively for clients' full experience in the response. They follow clients' lead in subsequent questions, using limited interjection. They are quite still and comfortably allow generous silences, trusting that the client needs time to reflect and will eventually say more. Practitioners describe and use words that reflect high empathy for and understanding of clients' experiences of their circumstances and, importantly, do not express judgement of the client for anything that is shared. The practitioner genuinely believes that the client has done the best that they could, given the situation they were in, with the resources they had (see Chapter 3: Connect).

BOX 5.2　PRACTITIONER REFLECTION. WHAT IS DIFFERENT ABOUT LISTENING MINDFULLY IN OPC?

So even when I was trying to be quiet and listening and nodding, my brain would be strategizing around where the client needed to go. But actually, to do OPC well, that has to stop. And so, I stopped it! By watching videos of myself using OPC I noticed that when I really listen mindfully I create more space for the participant to generate their own thoughts and insights about what's happening – that's really powerful from their perspective, but also for the whole invention itself. It obviously means you're really listening rather than pretending to listen. When I did this, of course, the idea I had initially had in my head actually isn't where the session went. Where it went was a much more successful, more appropriate place for it to go, from the family's perspective. Listening mindfully feels different. It feels more at peace with the situation, and I'm more able to elicit something extremely positive from the participant's point of view. (Catherine)

THRESHOLD CONCEPT #2: MEANINGFUL GOALS ARE WHEN DREAMS COME TRUE, RATHER THAN PROBLEMS MINIMISED

BOX 5.3　ILLUSTRATIVE CASE. MEET CATHY

Cathy is a 40-year-old woman who was diagnosed with multiple sclerosis five years ago. She works in a daycare centre for preschool children and has two children of her own, aged six and eight. Her husband is supportive but does not contribute much to daily chores around the house. Cathy is struggling to manage her fatigue. She is usually exhausted after her day at work and does not have enough energy to prepare nutritious meals for her family. She would like to be more involved with her children's activities but must leave this to her husband to co-ordinate as she is too tired. She feels that she is missing out on being a part of their lives. She also has recently started to have difficulty sleeping through the night. The video footage of this case highlights how Fiona coaches Cathy toward solutions by helping her to identify her aspirational goals, rather than by analysing her problems.

What are meaningful goals?

Goals in OPC reflect clients' hopes for a preferred future and emerge from a conversation about how a client wants things to be and what is most important to them right now (see Chapter 3). In the case of Cathy, playing with her children reflects her desire to be a "fun mum" and is a highly valued goal for her. Fiona seeks to enable Cathy's occupational performance and participation in life situations as efficiently and enduringly as possible, hence Cathy's goal directly reflects 'real world' changes. Fiona guides Cathy to describe what playing with her children would look like; that is, to express her goal as a specific activity in a specific context.

 Watch how Fiona interviews Cathy to identify what is most meaningful to her right now, expressed as engaging in a specific activity, in a specific context.

 As you watch, think about:

- What types of questions does Fiona ask Cathy to help her to identify what is most important?
- List the different ways that Cathy's goal is formulated and note how Fiona guides Cathy to describe the occupational performance that Cathy wants to participate in differently despite her MS.
- What effect do you observe on Cathy as Fiona guides her to express her goal as a specific activity in a specific context?

Initiating goal conversations in this way can be daunting to some practitioners, as clients regularly describe 'bigger picture' aspirations than rehabilitation practitioners have historically addressed. Aspirational goals (as opposed to problem-mitigation or 'realistic' goals) are also more likely to cross professional boundaries given that life's situations involve complex interacting systems. Practitioners can unwittingly guide clients toward more restrained expressions of goals (Levack, Dean, Mcpherson, & Siegert, 2006), yet goals that reflect the full complexity of what is most meaningful to someone *in this moment* are highly motivating, hence client's clarity, creativity, and striving become activated. Progress towards seemingly optimistic goals often happens quickly, irrespective of impairments. In the case of Cathy, Cathy is aware her fatigue is a barrier to spending time with her children and feels stuck in resolving this. She knows that fatigue will continue to be a problem as her MS progresses, and this knowledge weighs heavily on her. A problem-oriented goal for Cathy would be to minimise or manage her fatigue better but, using OPC, Fiona did not lead Cathy in this direction. Instead, Fiona drew Cathy's attention to what she values (her children) and dreams of (playing with her children). This goal stimulated Cathy's creative problem-solving and lifted her mood in a way that a problem-oriented goal of managing fatigue was unlikely to do. Importantly, this approach reinforced Cathy as a capable, resourceful self-manager of health and agent of change.

The power of motivating goals

Once Fiona invites Cathy to describe a goal reflecting her aspirations rather than problems, she can guide Cathy in quickly formulating what may initially seem a complex goal. This process is accelerated because the idea of what the goal will look like has been made clear. The practitioner can mentally 'declutter' other agendas (such as analysing and trying to 'fix' Cathy's fatigue) and listen more closely to what Cathy already knows about making her goal situation a reality. Through careful questioning and information sharing, Fiona is able to guide Cathy to a highly valued yet actionable goal (i.e., a goal that Cathy can actually influence progress towards) that has high chance of being achieved.

Motivating goals in action

When we observe practitioners who understand the therapeutic power of meaning-focused goal setting, we notice that they routinely open goal conversations with very open-ended questions targeting what the client values (e.g., *"What is most important for you right now?"*). The practitioner is patient, creative, and determined in rewording questions to guide clients to describe how they want things in their life to be, even with clients who present with low levels of confidence, expression, or physical and cognitive abilities.

☺ Reflect on how Fiona guides Cathy to identify an actionable goal, one over
which Cathy has some control but is still closely tied to her value of having
fun with her children. Consider a problem in your own life at the moment,
something you don't like or would like to be different. Write this down. Now flip
this to a description of an aspirational (the sky is the limit) goal. How would you
love things to be instead? Write a detailed description of this. It doesn't need to
be a SMART statement (specific, measurable, achievable, realistic, or time
limited), but it does need to be really clear and meaningful to you, and excite or
inspire you.

What do you notice is different in your enthusiasm to act on the aspirational
goal compared to your earlier problem statement? How might an orientation to
aspirational goals (rather than problem elimination) impact on your work as a
rehabilitation practitioner?

**BOX 5.4 PRACTITIONER REFLECTION. FROM PROBLEMS
MASKED AS GOALS TO ENVISIONING BRIGHTER FUTURES**

---

*You can write goals that are the reverse of the problem. You know, the
problem is identified and you are just saying you want to see that improve,
or you want to see that not happen. But to actually ask the family to
envisage what it would look like if that was no longer an issue, and then
pull out the language that they use when they identify that goal, it just
really frames it quite differently . . . The phrase that I use is "what would it
look like if that was no longer an issue for you?" or "Tell me about what you
want that to be like in a few months' time". Then families can quite easily
switch the language they are using, and the problem-focused stuff starts to
drift away naturally by doing that. For example, I had a family for whom eye
contact was a goal, which is a really component-focused concern. Knowing
how families value eye contact in terms of interaction, it would have been
tricky to say to them, "Oh, no that's component focused, let's not work
on that". So, instead, my questioning went along the lines of, "Well, what
does lack of eye contact interfere with?" And then the goal sort of shifted
a bit – the family was able to express that really, eye contact is about being
able to get the child's message across in relation to a particular request.*
(Catherine)

THRESHOLD CONCEPT #3: IMPAIRMENTS RARELY INFORM SOLUTIONS. ENABLING STRATEGIES CAN ARISE FROM ANYWHERE

BOX 5.5   ILLUSTRATIVE CASE. MEET JENNY

Jenny is married with two children, the elder of whom, Matt (aged eight) has developmental co-ordination disorder (DCD), also known as dyspraxia. A paediatrician recently diagnosed Matt after his school teacher and school-based occupational therapist recommended a diagnostic assessment. Jenny has noticed since Matt was about three years old that he often tripped and avoided ball play. Jenny still dresses Matt, as he seems to be incapable of getting arms and legs into the right holes. As he gets older Jenny is noticing more obvious differences between Matt and his peers, such as getting organised for activities, and she is starting to worry for his future. Matt has struggled academically at school, despite seeming bright and interested in his favourite topics: science, technology, and dinosaurs.

Matt has been referred to Fiona, an occupational therapist at the publicly funded Child Development Service which works with parents and their children (but not teachers). Based on what Matt's doctor and teacher have said, Jenny is under the strong impression that Fiona will be able to 'treat' Matt and 'fix' his dyspraxia.

The video with this case shows how Fiona worked with Jenny to identify strategies that enable Matt to be successful despite the challenges related to DCD.

What are enabling strategies for occupational performance and participatory goals?

The outcome of interest in OPC is always personally meaningful improvement in the clients' occupational performance and participation in life situations. When we consider the vast range of factors that influence an individual's occupational performance and participation such as motivation, task complexity, social attitudes, timing, technology, and physical support, to name a few, it is not surprising that attempting to minimise a person's body structure or body function impairments only occasionally features in goal strategies. For Matt, eating his dinner tidily with cutlery involves his sensory-motor systems, his ability to focus attention, the texture of the food he is eating, the type of seating he has, his motivation to eat without mess, responses from his family during meals, and so on.

A systems view, as portrayed in the ICF (World Health Organization, 2001) and the occupational therapy models presented in Chapter 2 (Law et al., 1996; Polatajko et al., 2013) that consider these kinds of multiple influences on successful participation, provides for broader possibilities from which effective strategies might be found than rehabilitation therapies have traditionally explored.

 Watch the video of Jenny and Fiona to see the kinds of strategies that arise when goals are occupational and participatory and when clients lead the development of strategies.

 As you watch the video notice:

- What kinds of systems (e.g., change to body structures or body functions, activity/occupation, environment) did strategies arise from?
- Consider strategies you use in your own life to complete challenging tasks. Which systems do these strategies mostly arise from?
- Fiona and Jenny agreed to work together for four to six visits to achieve Jenny's goal of Matt eating dinner tidily. How long do you think it will be before Matt eats meals more tidily using the strategies Fiona and Jenny discussed?
- You may have wanted to know more detail about how Matt's bodily systems were functioning than Jenny provided. How critical is this information to Matt and Jenny making progress towards their goal?

Mothers who had engaged in OPC to achieve child-related participatory goals reported strategies related to either adjusting the context around the child or engaging differently with the child (such as interacting more collaboratively) (Graham, Rodger, & Ziviani, 2013). The children had mild to moderate neurodevelopmental delays, much like Matt, yet none of the strategies identified as effective by mothers related to altering children's body structures and functions (such as strength, muscle tone, attention, or sensory processing) . The effect size for goal achievement in this study was extremely high (Graham et al., 2013). OPC is not alone in this finding, with numerous studies identifying factors other than impairments as key to improving participation outcomes (Anaby et al., 2013; Chang, Liu, & Hung, 2018; Willis et al., 2018). Consequently, assessment of impairments, a signature starting point of usual care in rehabilitation (Levack & Dean, 2012), is not undertaken in OPC. It is still important to be aware of impairments, but in our experience of using OPC, they are less relevant than traditionally assumed because they seldom inform solutions. Two of the main reasons for this shift in the relevance of impairments in OPC relate to the occupation and participation focus of goals in OPC and the emphasis on client-led change. Qualities of the individual, such as their abilities and motivation, are represented in OPC within the collaborative performance analysis process, but these qualities do not take precedence over other avenues for change. Instead, actionable change that the client perceives is achievable and likely to lead to goal progress is prioritised. In reality, what is often actionable is change to the social or physical environment, or the way an activity is perceived by the client.

In OPC clients are supported to achieve their goals over other agendas sometimes held by practitioners, such as developmental progression or 'quality' of a skill. Letting go of these agendas can be personally and professionally challenging, but doing so is critical to implementing OPC.

The power of a systems view for identifying strategies

A systems view of change enables practitioners to envision that multiple solutions could be possible to a given situation (Polatajko, Davis, Cantin, Dubouloz-Wilner, & Trentham, 2007). In relation to OPC, this requires us to see a life situation of the client for all of what it is, without assumptions, and then to question clients, listening for the simplest and most attainable strategies to improve on that situation. All factors influencing the performance context are viewed in relation to what enables success of participation in the life situation (as the client sees it) and how greater success, led by the client, could be engineered. The client's perceptions of the situation are part of the system of influences around successful occupational performance and participation. Thus, adopting a systems lens in coaching clients toward solutions facilitates a mind-set in which client responses to ideas about doing things differently are equally accepted and worked through.

A systems view of enablement in action

When practitioners embrace a systems view to enabling goal achievement, they open their thinking to a wider range of possibilities for change for clients. These practitioners are more likely to recognise possibilities for goal progress in clients' dialogue, as they will hear references to barriers that could be removed, supports or successes (bridges) that could be built on, or client attributes (such as motivation, stamina) that could be highlighted. Such practitioners are not hindered by the presumption that strategies are likely to emerge from bodies of knowledge which they hold as professionals or which are related to clients' impairments. Practitioners are unlikely to see detailed assessments of impairments as important to achieving occupational and participatory goals. These practitioners also assume less authority about how to solve clients' difficulties, since it is clearly clients who know the non-impairment aspects of their circumstances best. Consequently, clients' role as agents of change emerges more easily, particularly as collaborative performance analysis deepens.

BOX 5.6   PRACTITIONER REFLECTION. SURPRISING SOLUTIONS ARE OFTEN UNRELATED TO DIAGNOSIS

A mum that I've been working with has two boys. The older boy had been diagnosed with ASD and the younger boy was on a wait list for diagnostic assessment. Mum's big issue was how long it took her to get the boys to the dinner table. Basically, dinner was a shambles. They were often racing around. They didn't sit for very long. Mum was busy in the kitchen while also trying to get the boys to come to the table, and dad would just get home at that moment from work. Then the boys would, you know, ramp up, and mum thought it was all to do with autism and poor sensory regulation for the older boy, and potentially for the younger boy, too.

But, after questioning mum about where she thought the issue was, we worked out that it was really about this routine – about dad coming home and how excited the boys would get. They had the TV on and computer games, and when dad would come home he'd do rough and tumble play.

So during the OPC work, mum was able to identify that the TV needed to come off a little bit earlier – really, an environmental and task-related strategy. And she talked to her husband about some play when he got home that looked a little bit different and wasn't so escalating, like reading a book or doing a puzzle. So, in the end, the solution had nothing to do with the boys' diagnoses or symptoms or aspects of their medical presentation. (Catherine)

THRESHOLD CONCEPT #4: CLIENTS, RATHER THAN PRACTITIONERS, ARE THE AGENTS OF CHANGE IN COACHING

BOX 5.7   ILLUSTRATIVE CASE. MEET STEVE

Steve is an apprentice builder who received a knock to the head, resulting in a mild traumatic brain injury, while on a building site three months ago. Steve was unconscious for 20 minutes and was in hospital for seven days after the injury. He was living with friends at the time of the accident, but due to fatigue, headaches, and difficulty looking after himself, he has moved back in with his parents. Over the past month Steve's mood has dropped, and he has started to withdraw from his friends. He has not initiated returning to work and is becoming resistant to talking about work when this is raised by the insurance company case manager.

Steve's remaining symptoms, three months after the accident, include fatigue, headaches, and short-term memory difficulties. His parents have noticed that he gets overwhelmed quite quickly, e.g., if several people visit the house at once. Steve loved his job in the building industry prior to his injury, and on the weekends he was working towards a black belt in martial arts.

The video footage of this case highlights how Steve's sense of agency develops over the first two sessions as Fiona offers multiple opportunities to Steve to be an active agent in his recovery and in progressing towards his goal of returning to work as a builder.

What is client agency within coaching?

Situating clients as the agents of change is critical if clients are to take action towards their goals. Supporting client agency means allowing clients to take the driver's seat in their journey toward goal achievement. For some clients, this authority is naturally assumed, while for others, like Steve, the practitioner needs to respond strategically to encourage Steve to be the decision-maker.

 Watch the video of Steve and consider how you would describe Steve's sense of autonomy at the outset.

Describe specific signals from Steve that indicate how in control, or influential in his life, he feels. How does Fiona encourage Steve to be the agent of change despite his low sense of autonomy?

The power of client agency

Practitioners must believe a client is capable and creative before they will 'trust' making them more equal partners. Fiona actively works to partner with Steve in resolving his headaches and returning to work. Rather than directing Steve to seek a medical review of his headache medication, Fiona elicits Steve's assessment of his headaches, gives him suggestions for action, and invites him to make a choice about if, when, and how the medical review will be undertaken. At the next session Fiona again seeks Steve's opinion on the outcome of that review before moving on to his return-to-work plans. Steve is having difficulty with initiation and sequencing his thoughts. Fiona balances his need for structure and support with these cognitive difficulties against ensuring that Steve is the agent of change throughout their discussions.

With some clients, a sense of agency, authority over their lives, comes easily, and the practitioner's task during OPC is to ensure this sense of agency is maintained in the process of supporting client's recovery. For other clients, like Steve, a sense of agency is elusive and may be directly impacted by the health condition, such as the executive function impairments that occur with many head injuries. Despite Steve's limited initiation, Fiona repeatedly poses questions to him, inviting Steve to describe how he will progress from house-bound to working on the building site. Fiona persists in giving him opportunities to make judgements about his needs and decisions about his actions because she knows the power of agency is key to Steve acting on what is discussed and that it is closely wedded to his overall successful return to work.

Client agency in action

During her session with Steve, Fiona adopts highly collaborative, autonomy-supportive ways of engaging, being aware that she is in a position of authority over Steve from the outset and that Steve is feeling pressure from his insurance case manager and employer to get back to work. Sometimes during OPC the practitioner will need to 'do the partnering behaviours' before the client has taken up the role of active partner, but in doing so they convey expectation of partnering i.e., working together in which the client's contribution is highlighted as invaluable. This is a powerful technique in raising a person's sense of agency. Fiona adjusts her usual communication style to match Steve's cognitive ability. She does this by shortening sentences, asking more closed questions, and posing fewer, more concrete choices to Steve. Thus, Fiona optimises Steve's agency despite his impaired cognition and creates the conditions in which Steve can act on the steps toward return to work. Telling Steve what he needs to do (such as prescribing a home programme or an action plan) is unlikely to be effective, as Steve would be very unlikely to enact it. For the reader thinking of Steve's cognitive recovery, the coaching has also given Steve a challenging cognitive workout.

When you watched the video, what strategies did you observe that Fiona used to engage Steve in active decision-making? What other strategies occur to you that might also have been useful with Steve? What else might have been needed if Steve were more, or less, affected by his head injury?

BOX 5.8   PRACTITIONER REFLECTION. REALISING THE POWER OF LETTING GO OF CONTROL

Why am I so sure that the client will come up with a plan? It's taken time and practice for me to learn to wait. I guess gradually I've gained a deeper trust in the process of OPC, in arriving at a plan that the client owns. I've come to trust that I don't have to have all the answers. I've seen time and again this increased vitality in the client, a lift in their energy when I've given the time for them to reflect and decide on what action to take. I invest the time to wait because, so many times now, I've seen the client become more comfortable, and spontaneously describe using their ideas in other places. Family members coming up to me and saying, "what did you do? He's a new man!" I never got that before when I used a more directive, expert-who-knew-the-plan kind of approach. I used to like the structure that being the expert, controlling the direction of therapy, gave me. I still do like structure! But OPC has given me the structure to not need to impose structure on the client, if you know what I mean. (Ruby)

THRESHOLD CONCEPT #5: EXPERTISE IN COACHING LIES IN HOW WE ENGAGE WITH PEOPLE RATHER THAN WHAT WE KNOW ABOUT THEM

BOX 5.9   ILLUSTRATIVE CASE. MEET TRACEY

Tracey is the mother of four-year-old Jacob who was diagnosed with autism spectrum disorder (ASD) two years ago. Tracey and Jacob live with Jacob's teenage brother, who also has ASD (high functioning), and the boys' three-year-old sister. Jacob's father has recently left the family and is not permitted to visit. Jacob becomes immersed in watching the movement of string, picking grass, and throwing stones. He loves to climb. Tracey's current goal for Jacob is that he goes to sleep by 8pm. He currently falls asleep about 10pm, despite Tracey's attempts to settle him from 7pm.

After a psychologist has made unsuccessful attempts to work with Tracey to modify Jacob's behaviour, he has referred Jacob to Fiona, the occupational therapist, suggesting that a "sensory assessment" might help. The psychologist described Jacob as having very "low functioning" ASD and indicated that Tracey was quite rigid in her thinking and unable to implement any of his strategies effectively. Without contesting the psychologist's assessment, Fiona commences with an occupation and participation-oriented approach to the sleep issue using OPC.

What does it mean to be expert at engaging with clients?

In OPC our expertise lies in *how* we engage with people rather than what we know about them, despite holding specialist knowledge as rehabilitation practitioners. We discuss the place of expertise in OPC in detail in Chapter 3 in relation to the Share domain. We introduced the idea that sharing knowledge in OPC reflects 80% attention to identifying the knowledge clients already hold in relation to their goal, and only 20% attention to what practitioners might contribute as a guideline. We also introduced the metaphor of the 'info club' for those 20% situations in which the practitioner might offer specialist information. The expert information is sandwiched between requesting permission to share knowledge and asking clients if and how that knowledge could be applied. Remember, in OPC client agency is paramount at all stages because it enhances the likelihood of clients enacting change, rather than simply stating an intention to do something differently.

Moments when practitioners impart professional knowledge are particularly vulnerable points, when clients' sense of authority over their lives can diminish; thus, they are handled with care in OPC.

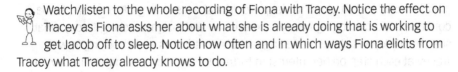 Watch/listen to the whole recording of Fiona with Tracey. Notice the effect on Tracey as Fiona asks her about what she is already doing that is working to get Jacob off to sleep. Notice how often and in which ways Fiona elicits from Tracey what Tracey already knows to do.

 What expertise does Tracey share that is likely to be helping this situation?

- What are some of the techniques or phrasing that Fiona used to elicit this knowledge from Tracey?
- Imagine how you would say something like that in your own words with the health population with which you are most familiar.

Later, Fiona does introduce some professional knowledge, to extend what Tracey has already been doing, such as ways of returning Jacob to bed without reinforcing getting up and the value of children initiating sleep alone. She does this by building on what Tracey already knows about getting Jacob to sleep:

Fiona: *From what I'm hearing Tracey, you have a lot of the basic 'sleep hygiene' strategies in place – clear, calming bedtime routines, no screen time leading up to bed.*

Fiona then links new information to Tracey's existing knowledge, while seeking Tracey's permission to impart new information before she goes further, with the following statement:

Tracey, the strategies you have described are many of the steps to better sleep that the research has also found to be effective for children with ASD. There are a couple of other ideas that have been identified as often useful. Would you be interested to hear about these?

Tracey nods but also seems a little hesitant, perhaps sceptical. She really feels like she has tried everything that any reasonable parent could do. Fiona notes this and continues:

One of the key conditions for children to get enough sleep and to settle themselves through the night is that they fall asleep independently – without an adult beside them. Does this sound familiar?

Again, Fiona seeks Tracey's engagement in evaluating this information and permission to continue explaining through her question. Tracey shares her familiarity with this information from the postnatal groups she attended with her eldest child. But she thought Jacob was too old to start that; besides, his meltdowns when left alone to sleep would wake his siblings. From here, Fiona continues acknowledging Tracey's experience and insights, asking Tracey what she already knows about managing Jacob's meltdowns and checking in with Tracey at each step on her interest in further information. Ultimately, Tracey and Fiona make a plan for Tracey to return Jacob to his room, without communication or eye contact, every time he comes out, requiring only that he stay in his room. Tracey also makes a plan of what she will do to support herself through this task, including asking her sister to be available by phone for support in the evenings and writing down the number of minutes between Jacob's visits out of his bedroom.

- At first, using this stepwise approach to sharing knowledge can feel artificial and slow, but it pays off. Clients are much more likely to apply that knowledge in their lives when they have been actively involved in choosing to hear it and deciding how it would be applied.
- Over the coming weeks, in your personal and/or professional life, notice moments when you *could* share information with someone. Try to catch yourself before imparting the information and apply the expert sandwich steps. Go one further, and ask first what more the other person already knows about handling their situation.

The power of expertise in engaging with people

Once practitioners understand that their expertise rests in identifying client knowledge rather than imparting their own, they can expand on their skills in doing this. It isn't always easy, and it is certainly more difficult with some clients compared to others, but it is rewarding to see clients solve their own problems. Clients often first meet practitioners with an expectation that the practitioner has the expertise to solve their problem, so first OPC meetings are often a time when practitioners respectfully direct clients to consider what they know, what they have already achieved, what could be tried next, and so on. Usually, client assumption of this role as a proactive problem-solver and agent of change grows as they themselves experience the success and power of this agency. As we develop our skills and confidence in coaching, clients become increasingly creative in finding ways to achieve their goals. But first we need to trust that clients in fact have expertise to contribute.

Expert engagement in action

When a practitioner has embraced the idea that clients hold much, if not all, the knowledge they need to achieve their goal, we see this in the way the practitioner talks about their expertise. Stories of practitioners' success in their work emphasise client achievement, creativity, and individuality rather than practitioner-attributed outcomes. Practitioners' professional self-esteem is no longer attributed to what they know about people or what they 'fixed'. Instead, practitioners see their competence reflected in clients' self-directed problem-solving. Practitioners less frequently offer information to clients and never offer advice on what to do, even when directly asked by clients what they should do. As one practitioner, Rebekah, put it, *"We all like the buzz of fixing someone else's problem, but the buzz is even better from helping them to fix it themselves"*.

 Remember the 80:20 guideline? How well do you think Fiona adhered to this? Maybe she gave too much information, even if she did used the 'expert sandwich'. What might the cost of this to Tracey's autonomy have been?

BOX 5.10   PRACTITIONER REFLECTION. WHEN CLIENTS SAY "BUT YOU'RE THE EXPERT!"

When I was first trying to do OPC and parents would ask me outright, "What should I do? You're the expert", I'd do one of two things – I would give too much information and not ask permission first, and sort of jump the gun a bit. Or, I wouldn't give any information, even when someone was clearly lost as to what they could do. With practice I realised that this 80:20 rule is a really helpful guide. It's not that you can't give information and it's not that you should give information all the time.

In an instance where they're saying to you, "I don't know what to do next; I've tried lots of things", I might respond with, "With permission, can I share with you what seems to have worked with some other families?" or "If it's okay with you, I'd like to tell you about some other parents who have done some troubleshooting on this in the past". It has often been another parent's strategy that I've shared, rather than some expert piece of knowledge that I had. Every now and then, some provision of information was definitely the right thing to do at the time. But that's been a really tricky thing to learn.

CONCLUSION

The five threshold concepts for OPC are concerned with the quality of therapeutic relationships, the meaningfulness of goals, adopting a systems lens in guiding clients' analysis, and seeing clients as the experts and directors of therapy, rather than practitioners. As with all threshold concepts, they represent potentially troublesome knowledge that can challenge previously (and often deeply) held assumptions. Yet once grasped, threshold concepts alter the lens through which we see the world. Next, Chapter 6 describes the research evidence about OPC to date, highlighting evidence of effectiveness with specific populations and contexts, qualitative knowledge of the experience of OPC by varied stakeholders, and, importantly, the limits of what is known.

REFERENCES

Anaby, D., Hand, C., Bradley, L., DiRezze, B., Forhan, M., DiGiacomo, A., & Law, M. (2013). The effect of the environment on participation of children and youth with disabilities: A scoping review. *Disability and Rehabilitation*, *35*(19), 1589–1598. https://doi.org/10.3109/09638288.2012.748840

Chang, F. H., Liu, C. H., & Hung, H. P. (2018). An in-depth understanding of the impact of the environment on participation among people with spinal cord injury. *Disability and Rehabilitation*, *40*(18), 2192–2199. https://doi.org/10.1080/09638288.2017.1327991

Graham, F., Rodger, S., & Ziviani, J. (2013). Effectiveness of Occupational Performance Coaching in improving children's and mothers' performance and mothers' self-competence. *American Journal of Occupational Therapy*, *67*(1), 10–18. https://doi.org/10.5014/ajot.2013.004648

Law, M., Cooper, B., Strong, B., Stewart, D., Rigby, P., & Letts, L. (1996). The Person-Environment Occupation model: A transactive approach to occupational performance. *Canadian Journal of Occupational Therapy*, *63*(1), 9–23. https://doi.org/10.1177/000841749606300103

Levack, W., & Dean, S. (2012). Processes in rehabilitation. In S. Dean, R. Siegert, & W. Taylor (Eds.), *Interprofessional rehabilitation* (pp. 79–108). Chichester: Wiley.

Levack, W., Dean, S., Mcpherson, K., & Siegert, R. (2006). How clinicians talk about the application of goal planning to rehabilitation for people with brain injury: Variable interpretations of value and purpose. *Brain Injury*, *20*(13–14), 1439–1449. https://doi.org/10.1080/02699050601118422

Nicola-Richmond, K., Pépin, G., Larkin, H., & Taylor, C. (2018). Threshold concepts in higher education: A synthesis of the literature relating to measurement of threshold crossing. *Higher Education Research & Development*, *37*(1), 101–114. https://doi.org/10.1080/07294360.2017.1339181

Polatajko, H., Davis, H., Stewart, D., Cantin, N., Amoroso, B., Purdie, L., & Zimmerman, D. (2013). Specifying the domain of concern: Occupation as core. In E. Townsend & H. Polatajko (Eds.), *Enabling occupation II: Advancing an occupational therapy vision for health, wellbeing and justice through occupations* (2nd ed., pp. 13–36). Ottawa, ON: Canadian Association of Occupational Therapists.

Polatajko, H., Davis, J., Cantin, N., Dubouloz-Wilner, C., & Trentham, B. (2007). Occupation-based practice: The essential elements. In E. Townsend & H. Polatajko (Eds.), *Enabling occupation II: Advancing an occupational therapy vision for health, wellbeing and justice through occupation* (2nd ed., pp. 203–228). Ottawa, ON: Canadian Association of Occupational Therapists.

Willis, C. E., Reid, S., Elliott, C., Rosenberg, M., Nyquist, A., Jahnsen, R., & Girdler, S. (2018). A realist evaluation of a physical activity participation intervention for children and youth with disabilities: What works, for whom, in what circumstances, and how? *BMC Pediatrics, 18*(1). https://doi.org/10.1186/s12887-018-1089-8

World Health Organization. (2001). *International Classification of Functioning, Disability and Health (ICF)*. Geneva: World Health Organization.

Chapter 6
Research findings
Ann Kennedy-Behr and Fiona Graham

Coaching has become increasingly popular as an intervention approach in allied health (Kessler & Graham, 2015; Novak, 2014; Ward et al., 2019). Using the Evidence Alert Traffic Light System of evidence communication developed by Novak and McIntyre (Novak, 2012; Novak & McIntyre, 2010), and based on the GRADE (Guyatt et al.) process where green represents high-quality evidence supporting the intervention (do it), yellow represents lower-quality or conflicting evidence (use cautiously), and red represents high-quality evidence demonstrating the intervention is unsafe or ineffective (don't do it), coaching has been variously graded in the green and yellow zones for children with cerebral palsy (Novak, 2014), with the most recent evaluation putting it firmly in the green zone for children with developmental disabilities (Novak & Honan, 2019).

Given the multiple methods of coaching that have been used in allied health (e.g., King, Schwellnus, Servais, & Baldwin, 2019; Ogourtsova, O'Donnell, & Majnemer, 2019; Schwellnus, King, & Thompson, 2015) and the overlap between different models, it is important in this synthesis of OPC research to be accurate and specific about the intervention names and terms used, particularly when evaluating the effectiveness of interventions (Graham, Ziviani, Kennedy-Behr, Kessler, & Hui, 2018; Ward et al., 2019). Some published studies have used the term OPC to name interventions when description of coaching procedures and elements are clearly distinct from OPC as described by its originators (e.g., Dunn, Little, Pope, & Wallisch, 2018; Foster, Dunn, & Lawson, 2013; Lum, Anderson, & Dean, 2018) . For a comparison of different interventions, please refer to Table 2.2 in Chapter 2. Further details about fidelity are provided in Chapter 4. This chapter summarises research that has been conducted on the effectiveness of OPC (consistent with OPC as described by Graham, Rodger, and Ziviani, 2009). Papers which have reviewed research on OPC but not reported original research (e.g., Alcorn & Broome, 2014) have not been included. Studies using OPC as described by Graham, Rodger, and Ziviani are summarised first, followed by studies reporting tailored or adapted versions of OPC.

KEY MESSAGES

- OPC has preliminary evidence as an effective intervention to achieve change in children's occupational performance and mothers' self-efficacy.
- Participants (both therapists and clients) engaged in OPC find it effortful but worthwhile.
- OPC after stroke can support clients achieve personal goals.
- Further research is needed into the use of OPC with fathers and caregivers from diverse backgrounds.

REFLECTIVE QUESTIONS

Part of evidence-based practice is to consider the characteristics of the clients described in research studies when deciding whether a specific intervention would be appropriate for your clients. Given this, consider the following questions:

- How similar are your clients to those represented in the research studies?
- Which similarities and differences (to your clients) might impact on your decision to apply OPC?
- What can you apply from the reported research studies to your practice?
- What might you change/do differently?

OPC WITH PRIMARY CAREGIVERS

The first studies published on OPC stem from Graham's original PhD research (Graham, 2010) and focus on the effectiveness of OPC in supporting mothers to achieve goals for themselves as well as for their children (see Table 6.1 for a list of original research published on OPC).

In an Australian one-group time-series design, Graham et al. (2013) invited mothers to engage in OPC to address occupational performance-related goals

Table 6.1 Summary of research publications on Occupational Performance Coaching

Reference	Research design	Participants and context	Intervention (and control, where applicable)	Outcomes	Evidence alert traffic light system
Ahmadi, Kessler, Hosseini, Rassafiani, Akbarfahimi, Khankeh, & Biglarian	Parallel single-blind RCT	15 mother-child dyads in control group 15 mother-child dyads in intervention group All children had cerebral palsy, living in Iran	2 groups: 1. 10 sessions of OPC 2. Control: usual occupational therapy intervention (neurodevelopmental treatment for child and parent education)	Significant improvements in occupational performance of personal goals and satisfaction (as measured by COPM)	Yellow/ Green
Belliveau, Belliveau, Camire-Raymond, Kessler, & Egan (2016)	Case study	1 male stroke survivor, living independently in Ottawa, Canada (stroke was 2 years previous to beginning of intervention)	10 sessions of OPC-Stroke	Significant increase in COPM results for performance and satisfaction	Yellow
Graham, Boland, Ziviani, & Rodger (2018)	Qualitative: interviews and focus group	4 physiotherapists, 12 occupational therapists in New Zealand	Participants gave their perspectives on implementing OPC with clients	Through OPC, therapists perceived they became better listeners; shared power with clients; raised some ethical dilemmas	N/A

Reference	Research design	Participants and context	Intervention (and control, where applicable)	Outcomes	Evidence alert traffic light system
Graham, Rodger, & Ziviani (2010)	Descriptive case study	3 mother-child dyads, Brisbane, Australia	10 sessions of OPC	Significant increase in COPM results for performance and satisfaction; positive qualitative findings	Yellow
Graham, Rodger, & Ziviani (2013)	One-group time-series	29 mother-child dyads, Brisbane, Australia	3–8 sessions of OPC (Mdn = 5); 54% of sessions were with children present	Significant increase in COPM results for performance and satisfaction; significant improvement in mothers' self-efficacy	Yellow
Graham, Rodger, & Ziviani (2014)	Mixed methods survey	Same sample as Graham et al. (2013)	Survey was at completion of previous study (Graham et al., 2013)	OPC took effort but was worthwhile; mothers gained insights about themselves; some indication of transformative learning	Yellow
Graham, Rodger, Ziviani, & Jones (2016)	Qualitative – analysis of coaching transcripts	Same sample as Graham et al. (2013)	3–8 sessions of OPC (Mdn = 5); same study as Graham et al. (2013)	Mothers were able to generalise strategies learnt during OPC to other areas; effective strategies were those typically used by all parents regardless of presence of disability	Yellow

Table 6.1 continued

Reference	Research design	Participants and context	Intervention (and control, where applicable)	Outcomes	Evidence alert traffic light system
Hui, Snider, & Couture (2016)	Multiple-case replication study	11 school teachers (9 female, 2 male), Quebec, Canada	1-day group workshop on self-regulation followed by 8 individual OPC sessions	Significant increase in COPM results for performance and satisfaction; significant increase in classroom management scores	Yellow
Johnson (2017)	Descriptive case study	2 mother-child dyads; Detroit, USA	6 sessions of OPC	Some increase in COPM results for performance and satisfaction; decrease in maladaptive mealtime behaviours	Yellow
Kennedy-Behr, Rodger, Graham, & Mickan (2013)	Descriptive case study	3 kindergarten teachers-child dyads; Munich, Germany	4 sessions of OPC with teacher + 4 individual play-based sessions with child	Significant increase in COPM results for performance and satisfaction; positive qualitative findings	Yellow
Kessler, Egan, Dubouloz, McEwen, & Graham (2017)	Single-blind pilot RCT	11 (6 males) in control group 10 (5 males) in intervention group; all stroke survivors, living in the community; Ottawa, Canada	2 groups: 1. 10 sessions of OPC 2. Control: usual care including allied health but excluding occupational therapy services	Significant increase in COPM results for performance and satisfaction; increase in cognition; decreased wellbeing and goal self-efficacy	Yellow/Green

Reference	Research design	Participants and context	Intervention (and control, where applicable)	Outcomes	Evidence alert traffic light system
Kessler, Ineza, Patel, Phillips, & Dubouloz (2014)	Case study	4 (3 male) stroke survivors living in the community; Ottawa, Canada	8 sessions of OPC	Only 2 participants completed study; Significant increase in COPM results for performance and satisfaction	Yellow
Kessler, Egan, Dubouloz, McEwen, & Graham (2018)	Qualitative – semi-structured interviews	Same sample as Kessler et al. (2017)	Interviews conducted on completion of Kessler et al. (2017) study	Coaching perceived to be helpful; some participants preferred a more impairment-focused approach	Yellow
Kessler, Walker, Sauvé-Schenk, & Egan (2019)	Conversational analysis of transcripts from RCT	Same sample as Kessler et al. (2017)	Analysis of coaching transcripts from Kessler et al. (2017)	Therapists need to be aware of possible power imbalance in goal-setting process	N/A
Lamarre, Egan, Kessler, & Sauvé-Schenk (2019)	Instrumental case study	1 female resident of an assisted living complex; Ottawa, Canada	8 sessions of OPC	Resident re-engaged in meaningful leisure activity; staff and family needed to provide extra support; minimum of 10 OPC sessions recommended for this setting	Yellow

for themselves and for their children (preliminary findings from this same study were presented in their 2010 paper (Graham et al., 2010). Participants ($N = 29$) completed the Canadian Occupational Performance Measure (COPM: Law et al., 2014), Goal Attainment Scaling (GAS: Kiresuk & Sherman, 1968), and the Parenting Sense of Competence (Johnston & Mash, 1989) at four time points (two pre- and two post-intervention). These three scales were used as outcome measures and were not a part of OPC. The intervention consisted of OPC alone (parents were asked not to seek other health services for the same issues for their child during the study), and the length of intervention ranged from three to eight sessions (over eight weeks), depending on when goals were achieved. To test whether the gains in occupational performance were due to the intervention and not children's maturation, the researchers compared changes over the same amount of time prior to the intervention as they did post-intervention. Results from the post-intervention measures demonstrated clinically significant improvements in both the children's and the mothers' occupational performance goals and satisfaction with performance. Mothers also reported significant improvements in their parenting self-competence. The reported effect sizes were medium to large. Interestingly, some significant improvements in occupational performance were noted at the second pre-intervention time point, i.e., before the OPC intervention had begun, indicating that goal setting alone via goal-related measures may have had an intervention effect. There was also some preliminary evidence that engaging in OPC enabled mothers to generalise strategies that had been successful for them towards other goals and that there was some continued improvement post-intervention for some of the goals.

The effectiveness of OPC in improving occupational performance has been supported by a small ($N = 30$) randomised controlled trial (RCT), conducted with Iranian mothers of children with cerebral palsy (Ahmadi Kahjoogh et al., 2019). The intervention group ($n = 15$) received ten weekly sessions of OPC plus usual occupational therapy intervention, while the control group ($n = 15$) received only usual occupational therapy intervention. For this study, usual occupational therapy consisted of neurodevelopmental treatment for the child one to two times per week for ten weeks and parent training on manual handling (how to move and position their child). As with Graham's study, the COPM was used as an outcome measure pre- and post-intervention. A Persian version of the Sherer General Self-efficacy Scale (Sherer et al., 1982) was also used to capture changes in parents' sense of efficacy as caregivers. Results indicated significant differences between the two groups. Compared to the control group, mothers in the intervention group demonstrated significant improvements in occupational performance of personal goals and satisfaction with this performance as measured by the COPM. Parental self-efficacy also significantly improved for mothers in the intervention group but not in the control group. While this was an RCT and as such a high level of evidence supporting the use of OPC, fidelity measures were not used in the trial (not available at the time) and the lead therapist had not had formal training in OPC, so some caution is needed in interpreting the results. These two studies, while different in design, provide moderate (yellow light) evidence that OPC can be an effective intervention to achieve change in children's occupational performance and in their mothers' self-efficacy. As parent self-efficacy has been linked to more effective parenting and positive child outcomes (Jones & Prinz, 2005), this is an important finding in light of the family-centred practice premise that the family is the unit of care, and not simply the child (Rosenbaum, King, Law, King, & Evans, 1998).

OPC has also been used with caregivers of picky eaters (four-year-old children). In a small (N = 2) descriptive case study conducted in the United States, Johnson (2017) found that OPC could support caregivers in managing mealtime participation. In addition to the COPM (Law et al., 2014) and GAS (Kiresuk & Sherman, 1968), the Montreal Children's Hospital Feeding Scale (MCHFS: Ramsay, Martel, Porporino, & Zygmuntowicz, 2011) and Mealtime Behavior Questionnaire (MBQ: Berlin et al., 2010) were used as outcome measures pre- and post-intervention. Following six OPC sessions which all included a family meal, both children demonstrated reduced maladaptive feeding behaviours as measured by the MCHFS and MBQ. One caregiver reported significant improvement on the COPM, while the other caregiver did not, however both reported exceeding expectations on goals as per the GAS. Limitations included the lack of OPC training and the very small sample size, but the exploratory study did demonstrate the potential of OPC in supporting caregivers in a novel area, adding to what is known about OPC with primary caregivers.

CLIENT STRATEGIES WHICH EFFECT CHANGE ARISING FROM OPC

Further research by Graham and colleagues (Graham et al., 2016) examined which strategies mothers identified as effective in supporting their child's occupational performance during the OPC intervention by way of understanding the mechanisms of effect of OPC. Videos taken of the OPC sessions in the study described earlier (Graham et al., 2013) were transcribed verbatim and analysed, and strategies were thematically grouped into either context-focused or child-focused.

Context-focused strategies found to be effective by the participants included mentally creating distance such as ignoring negative behaviour, physically removing themselves from the situation, better matching the task to the child's abilities, adding structure and routine, and adjusting their interaction style with their child. Fewer child-focused strategies were identified, but these included offering the child closed choices and collaborating or problem-solving with the child on goal-related occupational performance difficulties. Mothers in this study also reported that they tended to spontaneously repeat successful strategies in other occupational performance domains, indicating that some generalisation of learning occurred.

In their analysis, Graham and colleagues found that the strategies that emerged as effective were those typically used by all parents, regardless of the presence of disability. This suggests that coaching principles which involve the coach drawing on parents' existing knowledge and competence rather than providing specialised information may indeed be a valuable way forward (see Chapter 3, specifically the Share domain, for further information).

LIVED EXPERIENCE OF ENGAGING IN OPC

Mothers' perspectives

In a study which explored the experience of participating in OPC, all of the 29 surveyed mothers (the same participants as in previously reported study) found it to be worthwhile and recommended it for other parents in similar situations, but reported that OPC required effort (Graham et al., 2014). Participants were asked to complete a purpose-designed post-intervention survey which included both open and closed questions, based on interviews with mothers in a previous pilot study (Graham et al., 2010). Open-ended questions were analysed using content analysis. The researchers found that OPC encouraged mothers to take a more empathetic view of themselves and their children. Mothers' responses around gaining insight about themselves and their children led the researchers to suggest that OPC "may prompt transformative learning processes for parents" (Graham et al., 2014, p. 195). Transformative learning is characterised by a transformation in world view, where the individual is challenged to reconsider previously held beliefs through critical reflection (Mezirow, 2012) (see Chapter 2 for further information). The hypothesis that transformative learning may have occurred for parents in this study is consistent with mothers' spontaneous generalisation of successful strategies reported earlier.

While these findings are promising, the study was conducted with a small, relatively homogenous group of mothers. It is not known what the experience of engaging in OPC is like for fathers specifically or for parents from a different socio-demographic who might not be able to engage in the process or articulate their experiences as well as those in this study could.

Therapists' perspectives

The experience of engaging in OPC has also been explored from the perspective of those providing the intervention (Graham et al., 2018). In this qualitative study, occupational therapists (n = 15) and physiotherapists (n = 4) first completed two days of OPC training and then, after implementing OPC in their clinical contexts, participated in either an interview or a focus group three months later. Data were transcribed verbatim and analysed using thematic analysis.

A key finding was that therapists perceived they had become better listeners through using OPC. Even though the participants reported listening as standard practice in both occupational therapy and physiotherapy, they commented that through OPC, listening had become a technique used throughout the *entire* therapeutic relationship, not just in the early relationship-building phase (as they had been done previously). They also reported that using OPC had changed their overall delivery of service; for example, spending more time on goal setting and having fewer sessions with the child present.

Some therapists reported on ethical dilemmas that came with the power shift from therapist to parent which appeared to be inherent to application of OPC. For example, therapists "felt conflicted in empowering caregivers who could decide that their child did not require intervention because they [the caregiver] did not have sufficient concern with the child's participation in activities, despite substantial impairments" (Graham et al., 2018, p. 1389). Interestingly the central tenets of OPC which are occupation based were not reported as barriers by the physiotherapists, indicating that application of OPC is not limited to one profession and "may be useful as an interprofessional intervention" (Graham et al., 2018, p. 1391). Further research is needed to explore application of OPC across whole teams and professions.

OPC WITH TEACHERS

Two small, exploratory studies have trialled the use of OPC with primary school teachers and preschool teachers. In a Canadian multiple-case replication study, Hui et al. (2016) used a combination of a one-day group workshop followed by eight individual OPC sessions with primary school teachers (N = 11) to address goals related to classroom management of children with self-regulation difficulties. The COPM (Law et al., 2014) and GAS (Kiresuk & Sherman, 1968) were used as outcome measures, as was the Teachers' Sense of Efficacy Scale – Classroom Management factor (Tschannen-Moran & Hoy, 2001) at three time points: prior to the one-day workshop, at the completion of the eight OPC sessions, and eight weeks after the end of the intervention. Goals chosen by the teachers related to specific students, the whole class, and their own management style. Due to the small sample size, only person-based analysis was used. Of the goals set by the 11 teachers, nine reported clinically significant changes on the COPM performance score and ten on the COPM satisfaction score. Seven teachers' classroom management scores also improved to clinically significant degrees. Overall, findings indicated that OPC could support teachers in their management of challenging student behaviours in the classroom environment.

In Germany, Kennedy-Behr, Rodger, Graham, and Mickan (2013) explored the use of OPC with three preschool teacher-child dyads using a descriptive case study design. Concurrent with the intervention with preschool teachers, the children with developmental co-ordination disorder and identified occupational performance difficulties participated in a child-directed play-based intervention. The COPM was used as an outcome measure, and teachers were invited to set three goals related to the child in their care. Following four OPC sessions over four weeks, teachers' scores were compared to their pre-intervention COPM scores. As with the study by Hui et al., only person-based analysis was conducted due to the very small sample size. Clinically significant changes were reported for seven of the nine goals on the COPM performance scale and likewise seven on the COPM satisfaction scale (two teachers reported significant changes for all three of their goals while the remaining teacher reported significant change for one). Qualitative information provided by teachers indicated that although coaching was undertaken with a specific child in mind, teachers spontaneously generalised strategies to other children in their care as in the study with mothers by Graham et al. (2014). There was also some indication of transformative learning in that teachers reported viewing situations differently after participation in OPC intervention.

While the findings from both studies were positive and provide important information about the conditions for successful application of OPC, the small sample sizes and lack of control groups mean these must be viewed cautiously as evidence of effect of OPC. In both studies, the therapists implementing OPC had 1:1 mentoring from Fiona Graham but were not formally trained as training was not yet available; neither was the OPC Fidelity Measure (OPC-FM; see Appendix A). Using the Evidence Alert Traffic Light System (Novak & McIntyre, 2010), these studies offer only yellow light evidence for applying OPC with primary school and kindergarten teachers. However, the context-rich information gained through the two studies demonstrates the possibilities of using OPC with different client groups and provides a sound rationale for further research on the effectiveness of OPC in the education sector.

RESEARCH USING ADAPTED VERSIONS OF OPC

OPC after stroke

OPC has been examined by Kessler and colleagues for use with stroke survivors. Initially considered an adaptation of OPC (named OPC-Stroke) due to theoretical distinctions for people with stroke (Kessler, Egan, Dubouloz, Graham, & McEwen, 2014; Kessler, Ineza et al., 2014), research findings have indicated that the training, mechanisms, and processes were indistinct from those for OPC as originally described. Thus, the term 'stroke' has been dropped from subsequent description of the use of OPC with people following stroke in forthcoming publications (D. Kessler, personal communication, 23 December 2019) and in this chapter.

In a series of studies, Kessler et al. explored the feasibility of using OPC with stroke survivors, developed a protocol (Kessler et al., 2014), and carried out a pilot RCT (Kessler et al., 2017) with ten participants in the intervention group and 11 in the control group. The control group received 'usual care', which included allied health services (professions unspecified) but excluded occupational therapy. The focus of the intervention was on coaching stroke survivors towards reaching their unique participation goals. A large number of outcome measures were used, including the Reintegration to Normal Living Index (RNLI: Wood-Dauphinee, Opzoomer, Williams, Marchand, & Spitzer, 1988) and the COPM (Law et al., 2014) for participation and satisfaction; the Hospital Anxiety and Depression Scale (Zigmond & Snaith, 1983) to measure emotional wellbeing; the Goals Systems Assessment Battery – Directive Functions Indicators (Karoly & Ruehlman, 1995) to measure goal self-efficacy, and the Montreal Cognitive Assessment (Nasreddine et al., 2005) to measure cognitive function. The results of the study were mixed. Compared to therapy as usual, the clients who received OPC demonstrated greater increases in participation and satisfaction as measured by the COPM, but not on the RNLI. While both the RNLI and the COPM measure participation, the COPM measures participation in self-identified goals whereas the RNLI measures participation in a wide range of prescribed areas. Both OPC and control groups made progress towards achieving their goals, leading the researchers to hypothesise that goal setting (pre-intervention) may have independently had an intervention effect, which is similar to the findings reported by Graham et al. (2013). The intervention group demonstrated greater increases in cognition compared to the control group; however, they had decreased wellbeing and goal self-efficacy which the researchers attributed to increased insight into their condition, understanding of their limitations, and sadness that the intervention was ending. While RCTs are generally regarded as providing a high level of evidence, as this was a pilot RCT with a small sample size, the findings still need to be interpreted cautiously (yellow light) but provide moderate support for continuing to investigate OPC with people after stroke.

In a subsequent paper which reported on a qualitative study embedded into the original pilot RCT, Kessler et al. (2018) explored the mechanisms at play within OPC. Through semi-structured interviews with seven participants from the RCT, the researchers explored what was perceived as helpful or not helpful from the perspective of the clients receiving the intervention. Findings confirmed the importance of emotional support (now referred to as "Connect" – see Chapter 3) and that creating a trusting, respectful, and collaborative relationship environment was key to participants' engagement in the goal-focused problem-solving process that characterises OPC. Interestingly, not all participants were comfortable with the collaborative nature of OPC, with some reporting they would have preferred a more expert-driven approach focusing on their impairments in body structures and body functions. The researchers concluded that more research was required to explore how OPC with stroke survivors can (1) identify those clients who prefer a more therapist-driven or impairment-focused approach and (2) identify ways to tailor OPC for these clients. This study expands on what is known about the participant experience of OPC in the early stages of community life after stroke, highlighting the impact of timing and adjustment on engagement in OPC.

Kessler et al. (2019) further analysed the goal-setting processes observed in study participants during OPC, by applying conversation analysis to the transcribed recordings of the goal-setting sessions during the pilot RCT. Conversation analysis was selected as it allowed the researchers to explore not only the words used during the goal-setting process but also the interaction style, potentially revealing power dynamics between therapist and client. Findings from the study indicated that despite identifying as being client-centred, the therapists seems to have had the final say in determining goals. Therapists' perception of risk (client safety) and their perceptions of the attainability of goals influenced which goals they encouraged the client to select. Analysis of transcripts indicated that this was a subtle process and may not have been intentional, but that therapists appeared to restrict exploration of some of the clients' desired goals when they perceived these as unattainable. The researchers suggested that therapists might require explicit training in how to avoid restricting clients to 'achievable' goals. This paper advanced understandings of the potential for subtle and unconscious imposition of therapist authority during OPC which may undermine its effect on goal progress. Findings highlight the need for therapist reflexivity when applying OPC and key points for development in OPC training.

In addition to the series of studies carried out in relation to the single RCT, two other smaller studies have been published on OPC-Stroke. A single case study published prior to the completion of the RCT provided detailed information on the experience of engaging in OPC for one client. The findings were consistent with that of the larger study (Kessler et al., 2017) but also raised questions as to whether the client was participating primarily for the social contact of the intervention (Belliveau et al., 2016). This supports Kessler et al.'s (2017) explanation for the decrease in wellbeing experienced by participants which they attributed to the study ending. The participants seemed to value the social contact with the practitioner and conversational style of the coaching process. Further research is warranted to explore the contribution of enriched social contact as a mechanism of effect of OPC for some populations.

Finally, Lamarre and colleagues (Lamarre et al., 2019) trialled the use of OPC with older adults in assisted living in a single instrumental case study. In the goal-setting phase, the concept of personal projects (Little, 1983) was introduced as a way of framing the goal-setting process around expanded participation. Researchers found that OPC could successfully be used in the assisted living environment; however, it appeared that clients would need both family and institutional support to engage in the process given the constraints each could impose on client autonomy. As a single case study, the findings need to be interpreted with caution, but they do indicate potential for OPC to be considered in elder-care settings.

Kessler and colleagues' body of work on OPC with stroke survivors has greatly expanded what is known about the experience of OPC for other community-living people with stroke and the mechanisms of change within OPC that influence occupational performance outcomes. Using the traffic light system, OPC with stroke survivors is classed overall as yellow, i.e., tentatively positive but 'use cautiously' and measure outcomes to evaluate whether progress is made (Novak, 2012). Again, the breadth and depth of studies published thus far regarding OPC for stroke survivors provide an excellent basis for future research and sufficient detail for practitioners to decide whether it may be an appropriate intervention for their specific context.

FUTURE RESEARCH

As with any relatively new intervention, there is a need for ongoing research to confirm existing findings and explore other areas. The studies with primary caregivers provide moderate support but all were conducted with mothers, and no research has been published to date on the use of OPC with fathers. Another area for exploration is the use of OPC with clients whose first language is not the dominant language in their country of residence. As OPC is a talking therapy and relies heavily on verbal communication, it is possible that there are some limitations in its use with caregivers from linguistically and culturally diverse backgrounds or caregivers who have had limited access to education.

As neither formal training nor the OPC-FM were available for any of the published studies, an important area for future investigation would be into the use of these tools and ensuring that any research conducted on OPC is as transparent and true to the intervention as possible. Finally, future research is also needed that (1) expands the use of OPC with other disciplines, (2) compares OPC directly with a traditional consultative model with teachers, and (3) examines the economic costs and benefits of OPC, compared to other interventions.

CONCLUSION

The research to date on OPC spans working with caregivers, working with teachers, OPC being conducted by other disciplines, and OPC with adults (stroke survivors and adults in assisted living). With the exception of the two RCTs, most studies have been with small sample sizes and have not used control groups; however, they have provided rich description on the use of OPC with diverse populations and in diverse settings. Using the Evidence Alert Traffic Light System, the level of evidence on using OPC with primary caregivers and with stroke survivors is yellow, meaning moderate support, use with caution, and consider carefully the characteristics of the target client group before choosing to use the intervention. Broadly, participants in the reported studies found OPC to be worthwhile, and the outcome measures demonstrated significant improvement in occupational performance after the OPC intervention. Further research into the use of OPC with other client groups and the training processes and fidelity of interventions would strengthen the existing evidence.

The next and final chapter describes the impact that OPC and insights stemming from its implementation have had on practitioners working in a range of service delivery systems and populations, presenting several tools and resources they have found useful.

REFERENCES

Ahmadi Kahjoogh, M., Kessler, D., Hosseini, S. A., Rassafiani, M., Akbarfahimi, N., Khankeh, H. R., & Biglarian, A. (2019). Randomized controlled trial of Occupational Performance Coaching for mothers of children with cerebral palsy. *British Journal of Occupational Therapy*, *82*(4), 213–219. https://doi.org/10.1177/0308022618799944

Alcorn, K., & Broome, K. (2014). Occupational Performance Coaching for chronic conditions: A review of literature. *New Zealand Journal of Occupational Therapy*, *61*(2), 49–56. Retrieved from http://search.ebscohost.com/login.aspx?direct=true&db=c8h&AN=107827747&site=ehost-live&authtype=ip,sso&custid=s9679029

Belliveau, D., Belliveau, I., Camire-Raymond, A., Kessler, D., & Egan, M. (2016). Use of Occupational Performance Coaching for stroke survivors (OPC-Stroke) in late rehabilitation: A descriptive case study. *Open Journal of Occupational Therapy (OJOT)*, *4*(2), 1–9. https://doi.org/10.15453/2168-6408.1219

Berlin, K. S., Davies, W. H., Silverman, A. H., Woods, D. W., Fischer, E. A., & Rudolph, C. D. (2010). Assessing children's mealtime problems with the mealtime behavior questionnaire. *Children's Health Care*, *39*(2), 142–156. https://doi.org/10.1080/02739611003679956

Dunn, W., Little, L. M., Pope, E., & Wallisch, A. (2018). Establishing fidelity of Occupational Performance Coaching. *OTJR Occupation, Participation and Health*, *38*(2), 96–104. https://doi.org/10.1177/1539449217724755

Foster, L., Dunn, W., & Lawson, L. M. (2013). Coaching mothers of children with autism: A qualitative study for occupational therapy practice. *Physical & Occupational Therapy in Pediatrics*, *33*(2), 253–263. https://doi.org/10.3109/01942638.2012.747581

Graham, F. (2010). *Occupational Performance Coaching: An approach to enabling performance with children and parents*. Doctoral dissertation. Retrieved from http://espace.library.uq.edu.au/view/UQ:229057

Graham, F., Boland, P., Ziviani, J., & Rodger, S. (2018). Occupational therapists' and physiotherapists' perceptions of implementing Occupational Performance Coaching. *Disability and Rehabilitation*, *40*(12), 1386–1392. https://doi.org/10.1080/09638288.2017.1295474

Graham, F., Rodger, S., & Ziviani, J. (2009). Coaching parents to enable children's participation: An approach for working with parents and their children. *Australian Occupational Therapy Journal*, *56*(1), 16–23. https://doi.org/10.1111/j.1440-1630.2008.00736.x

Graham, F., Rodger, S., & Ziviani, J. (2010). Enabling occupational performance of children through coaching parents: Three case reports. *Physical and Occupational Therapy in Pediatrics*, *30*(1), 4–15. https://doi.org/10.3109/01942630903337536

Graham, F., Rodger, S., & Ziviani, J. (2013). Effectiveness of Occupational Performance Coaching in improving children's and mothers' performance and mothers' self-competence. *American Journal of Occupational Therapy*, *67*(1), 10–18. https://doi.org/10.5014/ajot.2013.004648

Graham, F., Rodger, S., & Ziviani, J. (2014). Mothers' experiences of engaging in Occupational Performance Coaching. *British Journal of Occupational Therapy*, *77*(4), 189–197. https://doi.org/10.4276/030802214X13968769798791

Graham, F., Rodger, S., Ziviani, J., & Jones, V. (2016). Strategies identified as effective by mothers during Occupational Performance Coaching. *Physical & Occupational Therapy in Pediatrics, 36*(3), 247–259. https://doi.org/10.3109/01942638.2015.1101043

Graham, F., Ziviani, J., Kennedy-Behr, A., Kessler, D., & Hui, C. (2018). Fidelity of Occupational Performance Coaching: Importance of accuracy in intervention identification. *OTJR Occupation, Participation and Health, 38*(1), 67–69. https://doi.org/10.1177/1539449217738926

Guyatt, G. H., Oxman, A. D., Vist, G. E., Kunz, R., Falck-Ytter, Y., Alonso-Coello, P., & Schünemann, H. J. (2008). GRADE: an emerging consensus on rating quality of evidence and strength of recommendations. *BMJ, 336*(7650), 924–926.

Hui, C., Snider, L., & Couture, M. (2016). Self-regulation workshop and Occupational Performance Coaching with teachers: A pilot study. *Canadian Journal of Occupational Therapy, 83*(2), 115–125. https://doi.org/10.1177/0008417415627665

Johnson, L. (2017). Occupational Performance Coaching for parents of picky eaters. *American Journal of Occupational Therapy, 71*(4). https://doi.org/10.5014/ajot.2017.71S1-PO4147

Johnston, C., & Mash, E. J. (1989). A measure of parenting satisfaction and efficacy. *Journal of Clinical Child Psychology, 18*(2), 167–175. https://doi.org/10.1207/s15374424jccp1802_8

Jones, T. L., & Prinz, R. J. (2005). Potential roles of parental self-efficacy in parent and child adjustment: A review. *Clinical Psychology Review, 25*(3), 341–363. https://doi.org/10.1016/j.cpr.2004.12.004

Karoly, P., & Ruehlman, L. S. (1995). Goal cognition and its clinical implications: Development and preliminary validation of four motivational assessment instruments. *Assessment, 2*(2), 113–129. https://doi.org/10.1177/107319119500200202

Kennedy-Behr, A., Rodger, S., Graham, F., & Mickan, S. (2013). Creating enabling environments at pre-school for children with Developmental Coordination Disorder. *Journal of Occupational Therapy, Schools, and Early Intervention, 6*(4), 301–313. https://doi.org/10.1080/19411243.2013.860760

Kessler, D., Egan, M., Dubouloz, C., Graham, F., & McEwen, S. (2014). Occupational Performance Coaching for stroke survivors: A pilot randomized controlled trial protocol. *Canadian Journal of Occupational Therapy, 81*(5), 279–288. https://doi.org/10.1177/0008417414545869

Kessler, D., Egan, M., Dubouloz, C., McEwen, S., & Graham, F. (2017). Occupational Performance Coaching for stroke survivors: A pilot randomized controlled trial. *American Journal of Occupational Therapy, 71*(3). https://doi.org/10.5014/ajot.2017.024216

Kessler, D., Egan, M., Dubouloz, C., McEwen, S., & Graham, F. (2018). Occupational Performance Coaching for stroke survivors (OPC-Stroke): Understanding of mechanisms of actions. *British Journal of Occupational Therapy, 81*(6), 326–337. https://doi.org/10.1177/0308022618756001

Kessler, D., & Graham, F. (2015). The use of coaching in occupational therapy: An integrative review. *Australian Occupational Therapy Journal, 62*(3), 160–176. https://doi.org/10.1111/1440-1630.12175

Kessler, D., Ineza, I., Patel, H., Phillips, M., & Dubouloz, C. (2014). Occupational Performance Coaching adapted for stroke survivors (OPC-Stroke): A feasibility evaluation. *Physical and Occupational Therapy in Geriatrics, 32*(1), 42–57. https://doi.org/10.3109/02703181.2013.873845

Kessler, D., Walker, I., Sauvé-Schenk, K., & Egan, M. (2019). Goal setting dynamics that facilitate or impede a client-centered approach. *Scandinavian Journal of Occupational Therapy, 26*(5), 315–324. https://doi.org/10.1080/11038128.2018.1465119

King, G., Schwellnus, H., Servais, M., & Baldwin, P. (2019). Solution-focused coaching in pediatric rehabilitation: Investigating transformative experiences and outcomes for families. *Physical*

and Occupational Therapy in Pediatrics, 39(1), 16–32. https://doi.org/10.1080/01942638.201
7.1379457

Kiresuk, T. J., & Sherman, R. E. (1968). Goal attainment scaling: A general method for evaluating comprehensive community mental health programs. *Community Mental Health Journal, 4,* 443–453. https://doi.org/10.1007/BF01530764

Lamarre, J., Egan, M., Kessler, D., & Sauvé-Schenk, K. (2019). Occupational Performance Coaching in assisted living. *Physical and Occupational Therapy in Geriatrics,* 1–17. https://doi.org/10.1080/02703181.2019.1659466

Law, M., Baptiste, S., Carswell, A., McColl, M., Polatajko, H., & Pollock, N. (2014). *The Canadian occupational performance measure* (5th ed.). Ottawa, ON: CAOT Publications ACE.

Little, B. R. (1983). Personal projects: A rationale and method for investigation. *Environment and Behavior, 15*(3), 273–309. https://doi.org/10.1177/0013916583153002

Lum, A. R., Anderson, M., & Dean, E. (2018). Using Occupational Performance Coaching in mild traumatic brain injury rehabilitation. *OT Practice, 3*(2), 29–30. Retrieved from www.scopus.com/inward/record.uri?eid=2-s2.0-85048705711&partnerID=40&md5=1f594d10f517739224
9ca4cb3b4784a6

Mezirow, J. (2012). Learning to think like an adult: Core concepts of transformation theory. In E. W. Taylor & P. Cranton (Eds.), *Handbook of transformative learning: Theory, research and practice* (pp. 73–95). San Francisco, CA: Wiley.

Nasreddine, Z. S., Phillips, N. A., Bédirian, V., Charbonneau, S., Whitehead, V., Collin, I., . . . Chertkow, H. (2005). The Montreal Cognitive Assessment, MoCA: A brief screening tool for mild cognitive impairment. *Journal of the American Geriatrics Society, 53*(4), 695–699. https://doi.org/10.1111/j.1532-5415.2005.53221.x

Novak, I. (2012). Evidence to practice commentary: The evidence alert traffic light grading system. *Physical & Occupational Therapy in Pediatrics, 32*(3), 256–259. https://doi.org/10.3109/01942638.2012.698148

Novak, I. (2014). Evidence to practice commentary. New evidence in coaching interventions. *Physical & Occupational Therapy in Pediatrics, 34*(2), 132–137. https://doi.org/10.3109/01942638.2014.903060

Novak, I., & Honan, I. (2019). Effectiveness of paediatric occupational therapy for children with disabilities: A systematic review. *Australian Occupational Therapy Journal, 66*(3), 258–273. https://doi.org/10.1111/1440-1630.12573

Novak, I., & McIntyre, S. (2010). The effect of education with workplace supports on practitioners' evidence-based practice knowledge and implementation behaviours. *Australian Occupational Therapy Journal, 57*(6), 386–393. https://doi.org/10.1111/j.1440-1630.2010.00861.x

Ogourtsova, T., O'Donnell, M., & Majnemer, A. (2019). Coach, care coordinator, navigator or keyworker? Review of emergent terms in childhood disability. *Physical and Occupational Therapy in Pediatrics, 39*(2), 119–123. https://doi.org/10.1080/01942638.2018.1521891

Ramsay, M., Martel, C., Porporino, M., & Zygmuntowicz, C. (2011). The Montreal Children's Hospital Feeding Scale: A brief bilingual screening tool for identifying feeding problems. *Paediatrics & Child Health, 16*(3), 147–151. https://doi.org/10.1093/pch/16.3.147

Rosenbaum, P., King, S., Law, M., King, G., & Evans, J. (1998). Family-centred service: A conceptual framework and research review. *Physical & Occupational Therapy in Pediatrics, 18*(1), 1–20. https://doi:10.1080/J006v18n01_01

Schwellnus, H., King, G., & Thompson, L. (2015). Client-centred coaching in the paediatric health professions: A critical scoping review. *Disability and Rehabilitation*, *37*(15), 1305–1315. https://doi.org/10.3109/09638288.2014.962105

Sherer, M., Maddux, J. E., Mercandante, B., Prentice-Dunn, S., Jacobs, B., & Rogers, R. W. (1982). The Self-Efficacy Scale: Construction and validation. *Psychological Reports*, *51*(2), 663–671. https://doi.org/10.2466/pr0.1982.51.2.663

Tschannen-Moran, M., & Hoy, A. W. (2001). Teacher efficacy: Capturing an elusive construct. *Teaching and Teacher Education*, *17*(7), 783–805. https://doi.org/10.1016/S0742-051X(01)00036-1

Ward, R., Reynolds, J. E., Pieterse, B., Elliott, C., Boyd, R., & Miller, L. (2019). Utilisation of coaching practices in early interventions in children at risk of developmental disability/delay: A systematic review. *Disability and Rehabilitation*, 1–22. https://doi.org/10.1080/09638288.2019.1581846

Wood-Dauphinee, S. L., Opzoomer, M. A., Williams, J. I., Marchand, B., & Spitzer, W. O. (1988). Assessment of global function: The Reintegration to Normal Living Index. *Archives of Physical Medicine and Rehabilitation*, *69*(8), 583–590.

Zigmond, A. S., & Snaith, R. P. (1983). The hospital anxiety and depression scale. *Acta Psychiatrica Scandinavica*, *67*(6), 361–370. https://doi.org/10.1111/j.1600-0447.1983.tb09716.x

Chapter 7
Practice in diverse service delivery contexts

Fiona Graham

Occupational Performance Coaching is an intervention, with specific fidelity criteria, as outlined in Chapter 4, and an emerging evidence base for specific populations, as described in Chapter 6. Interpreting and applying research evidence to our practice with clients requires consideration of the research evidence specific to the populations and outcomes reported, and the strength of the evidence given the study designs applied (Hoffmann, Bennett, & Del Mar, 2017). The existing research on OPC (see Chapter 6), including its limits, needs to be considered when decisions are made about implementing OPC in different service delivery contexts.

Threshold concepts are ideas that can be difficult or 'troublesome' (see Chapter 5). Like all threshold concepts, however, those of OPC cannot be 'unlearned' when working with a client who falls outside of the populations or stages of care in which OPC has been examined. The threshold concepts of OPC relate to relationships with clients and their occupations and have wide-reaching relevance across populations and health issues. Thus, it is unsurprising that practitioners have shared observations of effects with clients, which they attribute to OPC, when working with populations beyond those in published research of OPC. Evidence-based practice (EBP) is informed by the balance of research evidence with specific populations to achieve particular outcomes, applied in light of patient values and circumstances and clinical expertise (Hoffmann et al., 2017). Inherent to this widely accepted definition of EBP is a judgement by both practitioner and client as to how research evidence best fits their needs and context.

In this chapter we share answers to frequently asked questions about the application of OPC at various stages in the delivery of rehabilitation and education services and how engagement with clients might look when the principles of OPC are applied. The guidance provided is based on our clinical and teaching experiences, and stories and insights are shared by practitioners with longstanding experiences of implementing OPC in a range of practice settings. Rather than providing any definitive instruction, in this chapter ideas are shared for what OPC *could* look like in areas as yet uncharted by research findings, alongside examples of how some practitioners have revised aspects of service delivery in line with the principles of OPC. In this sense, this chapter is a meeting point between research evidence and 'wisdom from the trenches' of clinical practice. It requires the reader to be proactive in linking the ideas presented to their own experiences, practice settings, and judgements of what is helpful to their work while remaining cognisant of the extent of the OPC and related research evidence.

KEY MESSAGES

- Practitioners report that OPC, while familiar, is in many ways at odds with the system in which they work. For this reason, considerable mindfulness by the practitioner is needed to employ coaching strategies in direct exchanges with clients.
- OPC is an intervention, rather than a philosophy of care or service delivery model. However, the principles underpinning OPC, of person (and family) centredness, client agency (autonomy), and practitioner responsiveness to clients are relevant throughout the client journey, at all points of care.
- OPC has implications for service prioritisation processes, rationing of services, goal setting processes, service evaluation, reporting and documentation, engagement with other services, team configuration, and role definition.
- While resources to support these wider aspects of OPC implementation are provided in this chapter, a starting point for clinicians when enacting OPC is a clear recognition of the client as an active agent in their own change process.

REFLECTIVE QUESTIONS

- If each of the threshold concepts to OPC introduced in Chapter 5 were integrated into your service delivery, how would the client journey through your service look?
- What specific changes could you implement easily to create a service that reflects the principles of OPC? For the more substantial changes,

> what preparatory steps need to be taken before the service could make these changes?
> - Who are the champions that might support this change process for your service, and what resources need to be gathered?
> - What do you think are the limits of applying OPC? Where might OPC not apply in the client journey?

SERVICE DELIVERY IMPLICATIONS

One thing that surprised us about implementing OPC is how changeable our service traditions were once we had a clear vision of an alternative.

Rose, senior practitioner

Some practitioners attending their first OPC training question how OPC applies in their practice context, be that public, private, health, or education settings. Service delivery structures certainly affect the delivery of OPC (Graham, Boland, Ziviani, & Rodger, 2018), yet the opposite also appears to be true; the principles of OPC can provide an inspiration to practitioners for how things could be done differently. In the following section we present answers to frequently asked questions related to how various services and team structure can implement OPC and how they can monitor and evaluate their implementation; how the principles of OPC can be applied with people of diverse cultures and health conditions – including beyond current research (while remaining cognisant of current research); and guidance on communicating OPC verbally and in professional documentation. Each section stands alone, so the reader is encouraged to start with the question of most relevance to them.

How does OPC fit with service values?

An important question for any service is, "what do we offer"? Answering this question in relation to service values and outcomes provides a helpful touchstone when making decisions about what resources and training to purchase, who to employ, and how to word material that communicates to others what to expect from a service. Service values that fit well with OPC emphasise client empowerment, respect for client perspectives, and working in partnership. In Ella's experience, as a service leader at a regional, publicly funded community paediatric rehabilitation centre, supporting implementation of OPC is fostered at multiple points, the first being when employing new staff. Ella describes selecting people who espouse values and expectations that align with OPC, such as respect for the views of families, the importance of parent and child goals, and an interest in building family capacity from a focus on child and family strengths. Ella reports that while these values are relevant to the service's broader philosophy of family-centred practice, they also impact the extent to which staff will be able to apply OPC.

Central outcomes of services for which OPC is suited include achievement of client goals in the lived environment that reflect greater, meaningful participation in valued life occupations and situations. Julie, who is the operations manager for allied health at a community health service, commented that she and the management team decided to organise training in OPC for all the occupational therapy team, including management. OPC was chosen as it aligned well with the existing framework used at the health service. In-house training had the effect of upskilling the entire team and was also an opportunity for team bonding and creating a network of support.

From an employee's perspective, Mary explained that her first encounter with OPC was at a rehabilitation centre, where it was expected that all team members would use OPC.

> It was kind of department led at first, because others were using it . . . and it was an approach that was encouraged . . . [but] I was genuinely interested in it and I loved reading about it. It just was something that I [felt] was missing from my practice . . . like I really felt this totally makes sense . . . and it is so client led, and parent led and so positive that I just loved it from the onset.

How does OPC impact on practitioner time use?

The impact of OPC on practitioners' time use is often raised in training and research (Graham et al., 2018). OPC can take longer initially compared to more traditional approaches in which practitioners lead analysis and make recommendations. Practitioners have described OPC, however, as "saving time in the long run" (Graham et al., 2018) as clients become independent in self-managing situations more rapidly, initiate exiting services when goals are met, and less frequently seek services in future, when difficulties manifest in new ways (see Box 7.1). Additional practice changes reported by practitioners, which affect time use, include:

- Requests from clients for contacts to go from weekly to fortnightly to monthly as the clients gained increasing independence in directing goal-related action.

Practitioners report spending less time per case, but also sustaining a higher overall caseload.

- Greater use of phone call appointments, particularly after initial in-person meetings. This has particular implications for services that offer community-based visits at home, work, or school settings in saved travel time.
- Substantially less time dedicated to conducting standardised assessments (that were previously routinely administered) as a precursor to engaging in intervention and less time in writing reports. Practitioners report continuing to use standardised assessments and follow their usual report processes for non-OPC-related work roles.

BOX 7.1   ILLUSTRATIVE CASE. OPC INITIALLY TOOK MORE TIME BUT IN THE END SAVED TIME

In working with a multi-disciplinary team to implement OPC with people after stroke, Delis shared the following experiences of how time use changed:

Practitioners noted that focusing on client priorities and allowing space to explore their own strategies and experiences resulted in better 'buy in', which creates efficiencies. For example, a speech language therapist described clients as often having set ideas about using communication devices. Instead of advising them (that they were using it incorrectly), she allowed time for the client to explore different devices and to discover for themselves what would be helpful. In the end, less time was needed to find something that worked. An OT spoke about how she would usually do a cognitive assessment prior to OPC but that this was often threatening to clients. By exploring how things were going day to day, one client raised cognitive concerns himself and subsequently explored strategies that could work in his daily life without the formal assessment being needed.

Ella and Amelia summarised their experiences of the effect of OPC on time use:

We find that OPC saves the service time overall. The more we use OPC the more often parents find solutions and want to see us less as they feel able to self-manage situations. It's time well spent. Advising families on what they should do is not time-effective.

Similarly, a shift in time use when applying OPC is described:

> Nicole, who works at an indigenous health service as part of an inter-disciplinary team, commented that OPC saved time as *"the changes will be longer term . . . That is what I've noticed . . . I think if you're giving people recommendations then it might not necessarily work for them or might work for a week and then they'll lose interest . . . whereas if it's something that the parent has actually devised, come up with, practiced, fine-tuned it, [then] that's actually going to just be able to become part of their routine. And they'll have ownership over it. That's the beauty of it."*

Accommodating these kinds of changes to practitioners' time use required flexibility from team members, managers, and service structures. Incidental changes to time and resource use such as billing, car-pool timetabling, availability of phones, and private spaces for phone-based consultation assisted practitioners' implementation.

How can OPC principles inform first contact and triage?

Two services reported adopting OPC-informed triage processes to prioritise client engagement over client's health conditions, impairments, or disability issue (see Box 7.2). These examples illustrate approaches to service design, inspired by OPC, that, in the practitioner's experiences, heighten client engagement in the therapeutic process and minimise unproductive time for clients and practitioners.

BOX 7.2   ILLUSTRATIVE CASE. AN OPC-FRAMED PHONE CALL TO TRIAGE NEW REFERRALS IMPROVED CLIENT ENGAGEMENT

The local public health service in which Ella worked had a waitlist in excess of six months for children aged three and over. They had had a criterion-based triage system in place for several years but, aside from identifying urgent cases, it hadn't helped to provide the right service at the right time for many families. Ella's team trialled offering an initial OPC session at the time of referral with the option of a phone call format, focusing on family priorities and coaching parents through reflection, insight, and decision-making at that point. Distinctive from previous attempts, the team viewed this phone contact as therapy and attempted to employ the principles of OPC. They engaged families in envisioning goals and making choices on specific actions they could take.

> Ella reflects: *Through this initial OPC contact we are engaging with families at a time that their focus on the issue they were referred for is high. It also allows us to refer families to other more appropriate services if this is needed, rather than their waiting six months to find we don't have what they need. In the past when we tried offering a phone call at the time of referral, we were gathering information about problems in order for us to decide how urgent the case was. This led to a long list of problems that we could not then address, which left families very unsatisfied and still waiting for therapy. Now that the phone call is therapy, we are taking a more individualised approach to triaging cases while also offering service much more promptly, albeit just one session.*

By presenting an argument to their managers that the initial phone call was 'therapy', the team had it included in their service's funding metrics, thus dramatically reducing their wait-to-treatment times.

Similarly, in two private, user-pays services, Alice, Ameisha, and Bee describe how they have adjusted their intake procedures to allow for in-depth goal setting at the initial phone contact, which like Ella, they view *as therapy*. This phone session can take up to an hour thus needs to be accounted for in billing for practitioners' time. Rather than charging clients directly for this phone call, they integrate the cost for their time into the hourly rate if families decide to engage further in a course of therapy.

How might OPC affect team structures?

Research indicates that the distribution of roles and responsibilities between team members affects implementation of OPC. Multi-disciplinary team (MDT) structures are those in which there is limited or no overlap between professional roles and activities, often with distinct profession-specific goals (see Figure 7.1). Inter-disciplinary teams (IDT) typically have some degree of sharing of role scope and skills between health professionals, alongside retention of some

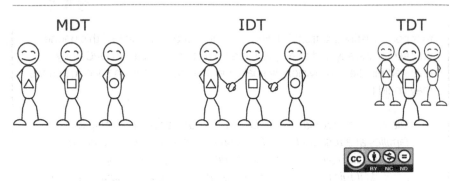

Figure 7.1 Multi-disciplinary (MDT), inter-disciplinary (IDT), and trans-disciplinary (TDT) team structures influence the application of Occupational Performance Coaching

Source: Figure 1.1 Three enabling domains of Occupational Performance Coaching. First published Graham, F. (2020), Occupational Performance Coaching Resources. Retrieved from www.otago.ac.nz/opc (29/01/2020). This work is licensed under a Creative Commons Attribution-NonCommercial-NoDerivatives 4.0 International License. University of Otago. Reprinted with permission.

profession-specific roles. Trans-disciplinary teams (TDT) are those in which there is a high degree of crossover in roles and skills between professions, sometimes referred to as case-management or key worker rehabilitation teams. IDTs and TDTs are often associated with better patient outcomes and higher patient satisfaction but are less common than MDTs (Ariss et al., 2015; Dean & Ballinger, 2012).

Practitioners describe how the implementation of OPC across the whole of service seems to work better using inter-disciplinary or trans-disciplinary team structures (Graham et al., 2018). Two features of OPC are routinely raised as challenging MDT structures: client-led, occupation and participation-focused goal setting, and collaborative performance analysis, in which clients' lead exploration of the dynamic systems influencing goal achievement. When clients are invited to describe their priorities in life situations at home, at school, at work, or in the community, the desired outcomes described rarely fall neatly into the body structures and body functions around which professions are historically organised. In addition, supporting the achievement of the contextually dependent, socially involved life situations raised by clients often requires either no expertise in body structures and body functions, or expertise that crosses multiple professional domains but applies to a single life situation. Users of OPC explain that the MDT model of profession-specific goals and interventions is not a good fit with these OPC processes, resulting in either duplication of intervention or redundancy of some professions around particular clients.

I've had to abandon [using OPC] where there's been another therapist not using that model, where there's one person in the room who's prepared to give the answers. If you ask an open question with genuine naïve curiosity, to find out what mum thinks, and you've got another professional going "well of course it's – da, da, da", then you're kind of a bit undermined.

(Graham et al., 2018)

Julie, whose service adopts an inter-disciplinary model, commented that while doing OPC in that setting could be challenging, it could also work very well provided there was understanding about the different roles. For example, the speech therapists might talk with the child while the occupational therapist engages in OPC with the caregiver.

Negotiating these shifts in roles requires planning, good communication, and perhaps most importantly, trust between team members. High levels of trust are a known criteria for effective trans-disciplinary teams (Dean & Ballinger, 2012), and this appears equally true in implementing OPC. Trans-disciplinary teams require clear agreements to teamwork, distinct role descriptions, low staff turnover, and a willingness from staff to (a) share their domain of expertise with colleagues and (b) expand their own scopes of practice beyond traditional professional borders. Managerial investment and support to create these conditions is critical.

In contrast to the unanticipated influence of OPC on the aforementioned team structures, some senior practitioners have described intentionally implementing OPC as a strategy to move teamwork towards inter-disciplinary models. Karen, a senior practitioner working in an adult community rehabilitation service, was the first in her team to learn about OPC. She saw the potential of the OPC processes around goal setting as a way to bring the team members focus together to a single set of goals. Karen shares an example:

When exploring what is really important to the client, is it actually driving their car, or is it accessing the community? I love that reflecting, reframing in OPC. We can assume their goal is learning to drive but in OPC we ask, is it the task of driving or what driving allows them to do? Then we can pull in the right discipline to achieve that goal, rather than all of the team going on working on several different things, that the client may be more or less motivated about. OPC gave clinicians the tools to have these conversations and now they are seeing higher levels of engagement from clients. Now staff want to revise our intake interview so that those more exploratory, values-based questions about what's important to them are asked from the outset.

A willingness to collaborate with the client in different team member configurations at different times in the client journey with a service appears to be a key ingredient and strategy in service-wide implementation of OPC (Graham et al., 2018).

Does OPC affect the overall amount of therapy clients receive?

When client agency, empowerment, and participation outcomes take priority over impairment assessment, monitoring, and remediation, visits from multiple health professionals are not necessarily helpful. Practitioners at a community child development service trained in OPC began to question the MDT team structure and, with this, the overall dosage of therapy that families were receiving. Practitioners became more attuned to the emotional experiences of parents during therapy (see Connect domain, Chapter 3) and gained awareness of how the MDT structure they worked within overwhelmed and confused many families. Practitioners began adopting a trans-disciplinary team structure for many aspects of their work, with one main practitioner visiting families but seeking support from colleagues as and when needed, thus reducing the overall number of individual therapists to which families were exposed. Practitioners acknowledged, however, that doing so required considerable trust amongst staff and managerial support.

How can the principles of OPC inform service delivery beyond researched populations and formats?

Practitioners often share with us ways in which OPC has influenced their practices with populations, stages of care, or formats not previously examined in research and we share some of these in the following sections. These applications of OPC reflect practitioners' enactment of the principles of OPC rather than strict adherence to OPC fidelity requirements. However, in the examples that follow we recognise the essence of OPC and felt that sharing these examples might help readers to better understand the central qualities of OPC through reading of their application in diverse ways. While practitioners need to remain aware of the boundaries of research evidence for OPC, we also acknowledge that practitioners use clinical reasoning alongside research evidence in deciding how to apply new knowledge.

OPC with at-risk infants and their parents

OPC has informed how some practitioners offer home-based early intervention for infants at risk of neurodevelopmental disability. Practitioners describe applying the principles of OPC to guide parent exploration of developmentally supportive play and self-care routines that are prioritised by parents, rather than taking a practitioner-led, developmental milestones approach. Parent concerns about infant impairments and abilities are addressed in relation to current daily routines and infant occupations (e.g., play, sleep, feeding, bathing). Using OPC, practitioners highlight parents' astute observations and responsiveness to their infant and explore alternative ways to engage in play or self-care that optimise infants' participation.

Infants identified as at-risk of neurodevelopmental disabilities are sometimes referred to developmental monitoring programmes by health services. Practitioners then try to engage with families who may not initially want any contact, may be wary of health professionals, and may be struggling to come to terms with a traumatic birth and newborn experience. Rebekah explains how she draws on the Connect domain of OPC in these situations, paying careful attention to the development of trust and partnership with parents during this stressful and often overwhelming period.

> *I work hard at developing that relationship. I know in OPC goals are supposed to be established right from the start, but sometimes that's a bit tricky. I might not be able to establish a really concrete goal for the first couple of sessions. There's a lot of grief to process because you know some families do go home from the hospital with a child who is has severe developmental impairment and may also be medically fragile and on oxygen. These mothers can be highly stressed and very tired mothers. There might also be other children at home, so it's really hard for a parent to be open to learning in that situation, or to actively engage in the problem-solving that OPC requires. Sometimes just being heard is the most important thing. So I focus on the idea of connecting within OPC – just listening and hearing where they're at, hearing that 'this is really hard for you' [mum]. And then you get to a point where the parent has more capacity to think about goals and next steps.*

Research evidence supports the use of coaching approaches with parents of infants with neurodevelopmental risk factors alongside other interventions that encourage sensitive, responsive parenting and enriched environments (Novak & Morgan, 2019). Here, Rebekah has drawn on her knowledge of these techniques learnt from OPC to enact these evidence-informed ways of engaging with families despite OPC having not been researched with parents of infants.

OPC in single-session contacts

For children of school age with moderate levels of neurodisability, many publicly funded services offer very limited support, if any. Informed by OPC, one service offers biannual, single-session review meetings, oriented around parent and child goals in daily routines. Using the COPM as a focal point for goal conversations and OPC as their guide, practitioners engage with families as leaders in deciding and acting on priorities and next steps. Amelia gives us a flavour of the direction OPC takes during these single-session meetings: *"At times the focus of meetings becomes the negotiation of goals between parent and child – that's where the therapy happens. At other times it becomes clear that the child's wheelchair needs to be reviewed, so we do that."*

While OPC has been evaluated with school-age children with moderate neurodisability, it has not been researched in single-session formats. Amelia and her colleagues are appropriately monitoring the effect of these single-session interventions closely through the COPM scores, reviewed six-monthly with families over the phone.

Tele-OPC

Delivery of OPC via phone or videoconference has been explored in two feasibility studies with older adults after stroke (Kessler, Dawson, & Anderson, 2018; Nott, Wiseman, Pike, & Seymour, 2019), both with positive findings that support cautious use until further, more conclusive research is undertaken. Here, practitioners share their reflections on delivering OPC via the phone. Amelia, working at a community-based child development centre, describes how they mix in-person and telephone delivery of OPC.

> We haven't made a particular policy about when to offer phone-based consultations, but we find that we work with families over the phone more often when using OPC. We offer families the choice of phone or in-person contact (at their home or in our clinic) and families differ in their preferences. Personally, I find that I deliver OPC a bit differently depending on whether it's on the phone or in-person. On the phone I can't see their reactions so I have to really focus closely on their tone of voice and words. I use a lot more clarifying questions and reflecting back to be sure that I have understood parents correctly. I need to listen much more fully over the phone but it does mean that the parent is really the one in charge, doing the analysis of the situation and making the choices.

Karen, working with community-living adults post-stroke, also finds herself offering phone-based consultation when using OPC. A key factor for her in this, she says, is feeling more comfortable with clients leading decision-making in OPC and not needing to be there in person to assess or decide on the 'right' strategy.

> Given the wide geographical area our service covers, even a few phone consultations makes a big difference to staff availability to work with other clients, so that incentive is always there for us. Using OPC via the telephone seems to work very well most of the time, with clients reporting positive progress on their goals.

Karen describes that key exceptions to the use of phone-based OPC delivery include when goals entail a safety risk, such as resuming cooking after a stroke, or when clients have significant hearing difficulties.

Adaptive equipment assessment

Several practitioners describe taking an 'OPC-informed' approach to assessment for adaptive equipment and housing modification. Although the decision to use a piece of equipment may emerge from any OPC conversation, OPC has not been researched in situations when the assessment for adaptive equipment is the central focus. Many practitioners describe to us that requests for adaptive equipment are viewed as distinct from requests for 'therapy', with the equipment itself often being seen as the goal, rather than a different outcome in a life situation. When equipment requests are viewed with the insights of the five threshold concepts presented in Chapter 5, the immediate question becomes, *What is the dream in life situations that the client would like to be a reality?* Ella acknowledges that she would describe their approach in this situation as 'OPC informed' rather than the full OPC process when it comes to equipment requests. Her reflections illustrate how the threshold concepts of OPC influence the way she and colleagues now approach requests for adaptive equipment or housing modifications and the effects she has observed:

> *While we need to share the limits of the public system's funding, it is a more thorough assessment than we used to do, that takes in a lot more information than simply a mechanical solution to mechanical problem. We listen carefully to find out the outcome the family are seeking in their daily life through the request for equipment, the patterns of how the family does things, and what is actually happening.*

Ella then describes how another OPC threshold concept comes into play, that enabling strategies can arise from anywhere, including from unexpected places: "*While this takes more time initially, the solutions we arrive at are often not initially obvious and don't always involve equipment.*" Ella adds,

> *Specialist equipment is an important option to have but when a funding application for a hoist or commode is avoided this saves us a tremendous amount of our time, and money for the whole sector. We've also found we have far fewer experiences of seeing unused equipment gathering dust when we visits clients later on.*

Karen describes similar shifts in practices when responding to referrals for equipment for adults with neuro-muscular health conditions. She relays the observations of one client who witnessed the services' transition from an expert based prescriptive approach to equipment assessment to use of OPC.

> *I have one client who jokes with me about the old days when his equipment OT was like having a PA [personal assistant] on hand to make calls, arrange for*

repairs, and drop off parts on his behalf. Using OPC, he obviously does all that himself, unless the funding agency requires a therapist to sign something off.

The client's easy rapport with Karen suggests that he is very happy with Karen's OPC-informed approach to equipment issues. Karen reflects on this:

Well, now he knows where and how to ask for the services he needs with his equipment needs, and where to follow up when the process gets stuck – he's not sitting around wondering if the OT remembered to send off the form.

Further research examining the application of OPC where adaptive equipment is anticipated to be a central component of care could inform how widely the experiences of Ella and Karen are shared and how specific practitioner actions affect client responses and goal achievement.

Can OPC work through interpreters?

The subtleties of language make translating OPC a complex process. Practitioners report that successfully using OPC through interpreters can require some compromises. For example, Ella described how at their publicly funded community paediatric service, they start with building a relationship with families by being more directive than would be consistent with OPC, yet being consistent with clients' expectations (e.g., recommending some equipment or exercises). Ella explains, *"Once the [trusting] relationship is established we gradually offer more parent decision-making, but it often doesn't get as parent-led as OPC requires".*

With lay-interpreters, it can be very difficult to know what has been communicated to families. Given the importance of how language is used in OPC, this uncertainty may mean that OPC is not the right choice in some situations.

DOES OPC TRANSLATE ACROSS DIVERSE CULTURES?

OPC has been implemented in New Zealand, Australia, Canada, the United States, Iran, Ireland, the United Kingdom, Germany, and Brazil and formally evaluated in Australia (Graham, Rodger, & Ziviani, 2013), New Zealand (Graham et al., 2018), Canada (Hui, Snider, & Couture, 2016; Kessler, Ineza, Patel, Phillips, & Dubouloz, 2014), Germany (Kennedy-Behr, Rodger, Graham, & Mickan, 2013), and Hong Kong (Chien, Graham, Lai, & Lyn, 2019). While findings from published studies on OPC across these cultures have been positive, there are many unexplored questions about the cultural translation of OPC.

OPC was originally presented in the English language with the majority of publication on OPC occurring in English. Some OPC resources, however, have been translated into other languages as interest in OPC expands, including French, German, Hebrew, and Mandarin. With translation of words comes the challenge of translating and adapting concepts across cultures (Beaton, Bombardier, Guillemin, & Ferraz, 2000; Sousa & Rojjanasrirat, 2011). 'Coaching' appears to be a difficult word to translate into several cultures, which impacts on explanations of OPC. Direct translations of the term coaching are often associated with sport, as in a sport's coach, or as a popular but unsubstantiated description of counselling which undermines the credibility of regulated, evidence-based health professions. In Hong Kong, Dr Chi-Wen (Will) Chien, who currently leads a study evaluating the effect of OPC with children (Chien et al., 2019), has used the word 'guidance'. Will explained that if he were to describe his use of OPC as 'coaching', *"people will think I'm going to offer hands-on exercise coaching"*. In French-speaking Quebec, Caroline Hui, who examined the effect of OPC with teachers (Hui et al., 2016), reported a debate among OPC trainees as to whether to keep the word 'coaching'. Some people suggested the use of the French word *'accompagner'*, which directly translated means 'to accompany'. This is very similar to a suggested German translation of coaching, *'begleiten'*, which can also be translated as 'to accompany'. Caroline shares an example of how she explains OPC to French-speaking clients:

> *I talk more about how we'll work together, and we'll figure this out together. You know, that kind of thing . . . I probably describe more of what coaching is than actually naming a model.*

Further description of how OPC is tailored for some cultures is presented in Chapter 4.

WHEN IS OPC NOT THE RIGHT FIT?

Some clients don't respond well to an OPC approach. While we can reflect on our use of OPC skills when clients do not respond well to it, for some clients, OPC is not the right intervention or this is not the right time for it. In OPC the acts of envisioning a different future to the current reality and taking risks to do things differently require a level of autonomy and competence that not all clients have at the time we work with them (despite our best efforts to draw their attention to their values and capability – see Chapter 3).

The expectation of some clients, that the practitioner will 'fix' the person and 'prescribe' advice, is difficult to move beyond and can be a significant barrier to implementing OPC. These expectations can come from a lack of accurate information about health conditions or evidence-based intervention options and may be more likely to manifest in the early days after diagnosis (Novak, Morgan, McNamara, & Te Velde, 2019). In order to move beyond this, it can be helpful to share information about the health condition and evidence-informed intervention options, one of which may be OPC. When offering OPC, it can be helpful to explain, in lay terms, what OPC is and why you think it would be appropriate. For example, a practitioner might introduce OPC to a client as follows:

> For the kinds of goals you have raised, I think a coaching method might work well. Would you like to hear more about it? It's called OPC and involves us getting a really clear idea of what you want to be able to do at home (school, work etc.) and then finding strategies to achieve your goal that really work for you/your family. Your judgement about what is working is a big part of finding strategies that work in the long term. Would you like to give it a try?

In our experience, clients are not interested in hearing a lot of detail about the approach at this stage but have expressed that they appreciate knowing that they will be taking quite an active role if they choose OPC intervention. Responding with empathy (as described in the OPC Connect domain, Chapter 3) to feelings of grief or loss can help clients to move beyond them and begin to consider their hopes for the future in light of the health situation. But not all clients will work through these processes within one episode of care or with the same practitioner, and OPC should not be persisted with when clients have clearly signalled this is not how they wish to engage.

Bee, who regularly uses OPC in her private practice with children and families, shares her views: *"some parents don't want the OPC model . . . they really would like the expert model and this needs to be respected"*. Bee goes on to describe how she does bring OPC into her work, often alongside other interventions and frames of reference:

> I think as OTs, we have a lot of approaches and models in our suitcases. I don't sit down with the parent and say OK this is an OPC session. Some of the principles are embedded in what I'm doing, and how I present things. Like suggestions for home, instead of saying OK you need to do this, this and this. I'll say well how do you think you could work on this at home? You know, just really working on that parent empowerment.

Occupational Performance Coaching also requires that clients have the cognitive ability to engage in sustained goal focused, reflective conversations. While scaffolding of clients' attention through simplifying language or the use of visual supports within OPC (see Chapter 4 on tailoring OPC) can help, for clients with significant cognitive impairments, OPC may not be the right intervention.

HOW SHOULD I EVALUATE OUTCOMES OF OPC IN MY CLINICAL WORK?

Outcome evaluation is an important component of any type of therapy, particularly when the research evidence is not well established or has not been applied to the population or context of therapy in which you are working. Given the focus of OPC on participatory goals, outcome evaluation should include the degree to which client goals of participation in the lived environment have been achieved. The COPM and GAS are commonly used measures of this construct and are recommended for both clinical and research purposes (Cusick, McIntyre, Novak, Lannin, & Lowe, 2006), although we suggest that only one of the two measures is necessary. Changes to clients' body structures or body functions, or performance of activities under controlled conditions are not relevant outcome measures of OPC, because the outcome of interest in OPC is always clients' personally valued goals in occupational performance and participation in life situations. Chapter 2 outlines detailed descriptions of how outcomes in OPC relate to the International Classification of Functioning, Disability and Health (ICF: World Health Organization, 2001) and models of occupation.

AS A SERVICE LEADER, HOW CAN I SUPPORT APPLICATION OF OPC?

Support practice change at all levels

Service leaders and senior staff are critical to any change process (Greenhalgh, Robert, Macfarlane, Bate, & Kyriakidou, 2004), no less so, it appears, when implementing OPC. Occupational Performance Coaching can be something of a culture shock to services that have previously taken a medical, impairment and therapist-as-expert view of their role. Strong leadership, which clearly supports a transition to prioritising client agency, as required with OPC, makes a substantial difference. Leadership support includes advocacy for changes to service design, a reconsideration of the infometrics that indicate quality, efficient services, and supporting staff if formally challenged by other agencies for not executing an impairment-oriented health system agenda (for example, if criticised for not formally assessing fine motor skills because of the child's diagnosis when it does not relate to a child's or their parents' goals). Practitioners at a service which undertook team-wide training in OPC described that knowing their senior managers would 'bat for them' enhanced their confidence in continuing to implement OPC and support clients' pursuit of their goals.

Mentor new staff

Ella, a service manager at a community paediatric service where OPC is widely used, describes a multi-component approach to supporting new staff to learn about OPC. This service has implemented OPC for several years and has adjusted service delivery formats and team roles to better fit an OPC approach, consistent with descriptions earlier in this chapter. This means that new staff to the service often have to learn quite different ways of working from what they have previously been used to, in addition to learning how to do OPC.

When new staff are employed, they undertake a broad induction process where they observe a range of different professionals working with children and families with varied health conditions, disability issues, life stages, and ages to see how the principles of OPC are applied. In this way, new staff learn more about the role they will take up, but also about what to expect has happened before and after they work with a child and their family and how to engage with their colleagues from different professions around a case. New staff are also provided individual mentoring from colleagues in how to apply OPC.

Alignment between supervisor and practitioner applying OPC appears to be key, given that for some, OPC is a substantial deviation from 'usual care'. Mary explained how she managed to get support from her supervisor for implementing OPC through sending her available research papers.

> I have support from my current supervisor who read the OPC papers I sent to her . . . and she has always been very [supportive] of empowering parents . . . So you know I have a lot of support at the moment but I have had a supervisor that didn't know about OPC . . . and it was a challenging supervision experience . . . It just didn't really work so well.

For established staff, having service procedures and documentation (as previously described) that are at least consistent with OPC help, thus enabling flexibility to modify things as needed to support implementation. Intermittent revision of training in OPC has also been raised as helpful. With the online OPC training becoming available, intermittent training will become an option for a wider range of services.

Practitioners have described the value of scheduled times for discussion of cases in which OPC has applied and peer-to-peer practice of OPC skills. Some services have done this within a section of existing team meetings, some have used videoconferencing for these meetings when working from different locations, others have used professional development time to go over OPC instruction and do role play practices of existing clients. Not only do practitioners feel this builds their OPC skills, it also gives them fresh insights into clients' perspectives when progress stagnates. Several services have described, including a 'celebration stories' section in team meetings in which case scenarios are shared where client autonomy or creativity in finding solutions to their goals has flourished. Celebration stories appear to provide helpful role models to new staff, raise all staff morale, and provide a reminder of the positive effects of elevating client autonomy.

COMMUNICATING OPC

What does written communication informed by OPC look like?

Our written communication as health professionals seldom captures all of our transactions with clients, but they do reflect and raise our attention to what we see as most important in our work. Written documentation that is designed to be shared with others (e.g., clients, colleagues, other services) convey not just what we have done, but the values that underpin our work. When reporting our work with clients using OPC, we want to convey our respect for and belief in client's agency over their lives and competence to achieve their goals.

Clinical casenotes and formal reports following OPC are oriented around client goals and highlight client authority, decision-making, and expertise. As such, OPC documentation emphasises client strengths, capacity, and resourcefulness. Significant barriers, difficulties, and uncertainties are noted when necessary, but these are not the central focus of written narratives, consistent with the main focus of OPC and aspired for occupational performance situations, solutions, and possibilities. A helpful indicator of how clearly client agency is conveyed in casenotes is to imagine clients reading them and coming away feeling understood and actively involved in their journey to goal achievement.

Casenotes

Practitioners' casenotes for OPC sessions mirror the Structure domain of OPC. Clients' goals are the central focus of casenotes rather than a summary of clients' 'problems' (e.g., bodily impairments, restricted performance, and environmental barriers) as might traditionally be the focus of casenotes. Documentation of hypothesised indirect inference about the causes of problems are absent (e.g., disordered sensory processing, attachment relationships, or problem-solving ability). Instead, OPC notes represent client-report of direct evidence of ability and opportunities to do something differently that clients' anticipate will support goal progress. Thus, the write-up of notes from an OPC session is reported as quicker by some practitioners. A format of casenotes following OPC could be as follows: First, the *occupational performance and participation goal* that was addressed is stated. Second, brief notes on *current performance* (at each session) are made. Third, clients' *preferred performance* beyond goal statements is described, reflecting the most meaningful aspects of client's vision of goal achievement. Fourth, client conclusions from the discussion of *bridges and barriers* are summarised, highlighting only key points. Notably, there is very limited or no reporting of what the therapist thought or did, with content instead focused on clients' words and action. Fifth, client-proposed *intended actions* are documented as specifically as possible. Finally, the agreement of if and when to meet again to review goal progress is noted. Tables 7.1 and 7.2 provide two examples of casenote entries following OPC sessions with an 11-year-old girl with autism spectrum disorder (ASD) and her mother. They are shared as examples of how some practitioners document their application of OPC but not as required reporting guidelines. We recognise that organisations and regulatory bodies sometimes have quite rigid reporting requirements that can be difficult to deviate from, such as when electronic record systems are in use. An OPC Casenote Audit Tool is provided in Appendix G, which could be applied to a wide range of casenote formats, including the one presented in Table 7.1.

While broader topics may have been raised by Leigh and her mother during the meeting, only information relevant to goal progress is documented. Major life issues such as marital separation, stand-down from school, or Leigh self-harming would all warrant mention because they would be *barriers* to goal progress, yet the organisation around goals is maintained. The same format for casenotes is repeated for each additional goal discussed within sessions.

Subsequent OPC casenote entries are usually shorter than initial session notes. The plan from session 1 is reviewed. Current performance, next steps, and discussion of how strategies can be generalised are all documented.

Goal statements can be copied and pasted into each entry provided the goal remains a priority to the client. If this isn't possible due to electronic record restrictions or handwritten notes, other strategies may be needed to maintain practitioners' attention to the goals.

Table 7.1 Occupational Performance Coaching casenote example session 1

DATE
GOAL *(Who, What Activity, Where, How Much, By When)* Leigh wears socks every day to school and for sports, supermarket, and trips out within four weeks.
CURRENT PERFORMANCE Leigh has not worn socks for 9 months. Hates seams, gets angry when she is made to wear socks. Feels tense, angry and excludes self from friends when she has to wear socks, e.g., at recent ice-skating party. Parents increasingly frustrated. Last wore socks 9 months ago when quad biking and they had to wear socks.
PREFERRED PERFORMANCE (Leigh's view, with agreement from mother): To be able to laugh with her friends; to be able to whizz around the skating rink in the middle with her friends; Mum and Dad to be happier with her.
BRIDGES AND BARRIERS **(Person** : Motivation, Knowledge; **Task** : Ability, Steps, Sequence, Standard; **Environment** : Social, Physical)* BARRIERS: Doesn't like wool. Doesn't like seams. Gets worried before putting on socks. She tells herself that she doesn't like it, feels worse. Feels like a vicious circle to Leigh and mum. Mum says she does not understand why Leigh will not wear socks. BRIDGES: Discussed differences in individual's sensory processing/sensitivities. Discussed seamless socks, rubbing fabric on feet to 'de-sensitise them'; Leigh notices that she can wear socks when she is distracted, e.g., when watching TV.
ACTION PLAN (Mum): Let Leigh lead decision-making about socks. Buy seamless socks for Leigh to try. (Leigh): Choose a TV programme. Put on socks five minutes into the programme. Keep them on for the whole programme for one week. After one week try to keep them on until she goes to bed. Practise breathing techniques in bed at night.
NEXT MEETING • Two weeks' time.

Table 7.2 Occupational Performance Coaching casenote example session 2

DATE
GOAL *(Who, What Activity, Where, How Much, By When)* Leigh to wear socks every day to school and at weekends and after school when required for sports, supermarket, and trips out within four weeks.
CURRENT PERFORMANCE Followed the plan but initially unable to wear socks. From second day of TV time, wore socks only for TV time. About fifth night, wore socks to bed. On day trip to adventure park with mum wore socks all day. Wearing socks for part of each day currently.
PREFERRED PERFORMANCE For Leigh to wear socks easily (keeping calm) without the need for TV/computer/ exciting trips and for Leigh to be able to wear socks to school.
BRIDGES AND BARRIERS **(Person** *: Motivation, Knowledge;* **Task** *: Ability, Steps, Sequence, Standard;* **Environment** *: Social, Physical)* BRIDGES: Mum and Leigh report that seamless socks help a bit and they think they might work at school. Making plans together (Leigh and mum) to tackle difficult problems is more fun than arguing like before. BARRIERS: Keep forgetting to do breathing practice, but Leigh thinks it helps. Mum is worried that Leigh might give up trying to wear socks after school.
ACTION PLAN (Mum): Keep letting Leigh lead decision-making about things she wants to be able to do (e.g., trying on new clothes, going to parties, getting off to sleep). (Leigh): Wear seamless socks to school. Wear other socks every day to keep practicing. To practise belly breathing and try some breathing apps.
NEXT MEETING • Two weeks' time.

A blank version of this template for Occupational Performance Coaching casenotes is provided in Appendix H and can also be downloaded and printed from www.otago.ac.nz/opc.

Communicating OPC to colleagues and partner agencies

Clarity in reporting clients' processes and outcomes when using OPC are particularly important for communicating how we work and upholding clients' authority over the next steps in their journey. While report writing can feel divorced from our real work with clients, reports are often the only way that those outside of the therapy encounter gain an insight into what practitioners offered and how clients responded. Reports are also often the last word about an episode or phase within a client's life, thus they can leave a tangible and lasting impression on clients and others connected to them. It is important, therefore, that formal reporting writing following OPC aligns with the principles of OPC – genuine empathy and respect, partnership, promotion of client agency and capability, and an occupational and participatory focus. Having said that, several of us have found that we write much less formal reports (i.e., intake, summary, or discharge) when OPC has been used (see Appendix I). Rather than enacting therapist-directed processes of care and writing reports as a matter of routine, we ask clients what would be helpful to them as they exit the service. Seldom do clients want a report of their episode of OPC. Although OPC is not a form of counselling, the value of a report to a client after OPC may be similar to that after receiving counselling or psychotherapy – not much. The highly personal learning processes that often occur within OPC are experienced by clients, rather than needing to be memory cues. When reports are needed, e.g., to referring agencies or service funders, it is recommended that these follow a similar structure to that described for casenotes, with client occupational and participatory goals as the central organising idea.

CONCLUSION

Implementing OPC into existing service systems can be challenging, particularly for practitioners who are alone in their attempts. True to their definition, the threshold concepts of OPC, presented in Chapter 5, can have wide-reaching implication for how things are seen beyond the intervention itself, such as service delivery design. In addition, many aspects of service delivery in relation to OPC have not yet been formally studied. Yet, several practitioners and services have addressed these challenges in ways that uphold the principles of OPC, including in areas of work that are beyond the scope of an intervention, as illustrated in this chapter.

REFERENCES

Ariss, S. M., Enderby, P. M., Smith, T., Nancarrow, S. A., Bradburn, M. J., Harrop, D., . . . Ryan, T. (2015). Secondary analysis and literature review of community rehabilitation and intermediate care: An information resource. *Health Services and Delivery Research, 3*(1).

Beaton, D. E., Bombardier, C., Guillemin, F., & Ferraz, M. B. (2000). Guidelines for the process of cross-cultural adaptation of self-report measures. *Spine*, *25*, 3186–3191. https://doi.org/10.1097/00007632-200012150-00014

Chien, C. W., Graham, F., Lai, Y. C., & Lyn, C. (2019). *A parent coaching intervention to promote community participation of young children with developmental disability* [Research Grant]. Hong Kong: Health and Medical Research Fund.

Cusick, A., McIntyre, S., Novak, I., Lannin, N., & Lowe, K. (2006). A comparison of Goal Attainment Scaling and the Canadian Occupational Performance Measure for paediatric rehabilitation research. *Pediatric Rehabilitation*, *9*(2), 149–157. https://doi.org/10.1080/13638490500235581

Dean, S., & Ballinger, C. (2012). An interprofessional approach to rehabilitation. In S. Dean, R. Siegert, & W. Taylor (Eds.), *Interprofessional rehabilitation: A person-centered approach* (pp. 45–78). Chichester: Wiley.

Graham, F., Boland, P., Ziviani, J., & Rodger, S. (2018). Occupational therapists' and physiotherapists' perceptions of implementing Occupational Performance Coaching. *Disability and Rehabilitation*, *40*(12), 1386–1392. https://doi.org/10.1080/09638288.2017.1295474

Graham, F., Rodger, S., & Ziviani, J. (2013). Effectiveness of Occupational Performance Coaching in improving children's and mothers' performance and mothers' self-competence. *American Journal of Occupational Therapy*, *67*(1), 10–18. https://doi.org/10.5014/ajot.2013.004648

Greenhalgh, T., Robert, G., Macfarlane, F., Bate, P., & Kyriakidou, O. (2004). Diffusion of innovations in service organizations: Systematic review and recommendations. *The Milbank Quarterly*, *82*(4), 581–629. https://doi.org/10.1111/j.0887-378X.2004.00325.x

Hoffmann, T., Bennett, S., & Del Mar, C. (2017). Introduction of evidence-based practice. In T. Hoffman, S. Bennett, & C. Del Mar (Eds.), *Evidence-based practice across the health professions* (3rd ed., pp. 1–15). Chatswood, NSW: Elsevier.

Hui, C., Snider, L., & Couture, M. (2016). Self-regulation workshop and Occupational Performance Coaching with teachers: A pilot project. *Canadian Journal of Occupational Therapy*, *83*(2), 115–125. https://doi.org/10.1177/0008417415627665

Kennedy-Behr, A., Rodger, S., Graham, F., & Mickan, S. (2013). Creating enabling environments at preschool for children with developmental coordination disorder. *Journal of Occupational Therapy, Schools, & Early Intervention*, *6*(4), 301–313. https://doi.org/10.1080/19411243.2013.860760

Kessler, D., Dawson, D., & Anderson, N. (2018, October). *Is Occupational Performance Coaching for stroke survivors delivered via telerehabiitation (tele-OPC-stroke) feasible and acceptable to recipients?* Poster presented at the 11th World Stroke Congress, Montreal, CA.

Kessler, D., Ineza, I., Patel, H., Phillips, M., & Dubouloz, C. (2014). Occupational Performance Coaching adapted for stroke survivors (OPC-Stroke): A feasibility evaluation. *Physical & Occupational Therapy in Geriatrics*, *32*(1), 42–57. https://doi.org/10.3109/02703181.2013.873845

Nott, M., Wiseman, L., Pike, S., & Seymour, T. (2019, July). *Stroke self-management supported by Occupational Therapy Coaching in rural New South Wales*. Paper presented at the Occupational Therapy Australia 28th National Conference and Exhibition: "Together Towards Tomorrow", Sydney, AU.

Novak, I., & Morgan, C. (2019). High-risk follow-up: Early intervention and rehabilitation. In *Handbook of clinical neurology series* (1st ed., Vol. 162, pp. 483–510). Amsterdam, NL: Elsevier.

Novak, I., Morgan, C., McNamara, L., & Te Velde, A. (2019). Best practice guidelines for communicating to parents the diagnosis of disability. *Early Human Development*, *139*, 104841. https://doi.org/10.1016/j.earlhumdev.2019.104841

Sousa, V. D., & Rojjanasrirat, W. (2011). Translation, adaptation and validation of instruments or scales for use in cross-cultural health care research: A clear and user-friendly guideline. *Journal of Evaluation in Clinical Practice*, *17*(2), 268–274. https://doi.org/10.1111/j.1365-2753.2010.01434.x

World Health Organization. (2001). *International Classification of Functioning, Disability and Health (ICF)*. Geneva: World Health Organization.

Afterword

Fiona Graham, Ann Kennedy-Behr, and Jenny Ziviani

We encourage you to approach the ideas presented in this book open to the possibilities for your work that they offer. Some ideas will have been familiar to you. We hope these affirm to you the value of what you already know and your wisdom in already discovering this information. Some ideas might challenge your current ways of practicing, your idea of what it means to do your job well, or what the system that you work in should look like. Challenging ideas can lead to growth for individuals and organisations. Often when we really question why we do things a particular way, there is more flexibility about how we work than it initially seemed. We also hope that some ideas in this book provide you with practical information and strategies for how to do things differently to achieve even better outcomes for the clients with whom you work. Often our greatest hurdle is clarifying our vision of what is possible. Dream big.

Appendix A: Occupational Performance Coaching Fidelity Measure (OPC-FM)

SCALE DESCRIPTORS AND RATING GUIDE

The Occupational Performance Coaching Fidelity Measure (OPC-FM) reflects raters' perceptions of the occurrence and quality of therapist and client behaviours described in OPC-FM items, with general instruction provided in Table A.1 ('OPC-FM generic scale descriptors') and item-specific instruction provided in Table A.2 ('OPC-FM item descriptor and detailed rating guide'). Non-occurrence of therapist behaviour is indicated by a score of 0. Levels 1 to 3 indicate that the item occurred in the coaching *and* the quality of the therapist behaviour. Quality refers to how skilfully the therapist applies the OPC behaviour in the context of the particular therapist-client context. Distinguishing items are rated in the same way as other items, with scoring reversed when scores are being summated. Definitions of each level of the scale are provided in Table A.1 'OPC-FM generic scale descriptors'. Scores can be transferred to the summary score sheet (Table A.3) to facilitate scoring.

In brief, a score of:

0   indicates that there was no evidence of the item behaviour.
1   indicates that there was poor use of a behaviour to the extent that it is very unlikely that a therapeutic effect toward goal achievement will occur.
2   indicates that moderate evidence of the behaviour was observed, however some opportunities to extend the use of the item behaviour were missed, to the extent that goal progress is likely to be limited.
3   indicates that almost all opportunities to apply the item were taken and fully utilised, to the extent that they are likely to substantially impact sustainable, goal-related actions and, thus, substantially influence goal achievement.

Table A.1 OPC-FM generic scale descriptors

Score	Therapist items	Client items
0	Therapist *does not demonstrate* the behaviour. The behaviour is not observed.	Client *does not demonstrate* or express the behaviour related to the item. There is no evidence of the intended response to the relevant therapist behaviours.
1	Therapist demonstrates the behaviour and the quality of behaviour is *low*. An attempt at the behaviour by the therapist was observed, but the attempt did not elicit (or is not expected to elicit) the intended response from the client. The behaviour may have been ambiguous, incomplete, or poorly timed.	The client exhibits or expresses the behaviour to a *low level*. There is some but very limited evidence that the client is responding as intended to the relevant therapist behaviours but responses are so weak that there is likely to be no sustained impact on goal achievement.
2	Therapist demonstrates the behaviour and quality of behaviour is *moderate*. An attempt at the behaviour was observed but with only *moderate accuracy* in relation to client's needs. A response from the client was observed but the rater perceives that a stronger response could have been elicited.	The client exhibits or expresses the behaviour to a *moderate level*, irrespective of the quality of therapist behaviour. There is moderate evidence that the client is responding as intended to the relevant therapist behaviours but a more overt response is desirable. There is likely to be a moderate impact on goal achievement but the full response was not apparent.
3	Therapist demonstrates the behaviour and the quality of the behaviour is *high*. An attempt at the behaviour by the therapist was observed which would normally be expected to elicited a strong response from the client, irrespective of whether it actually elicits a strong response.	The client exhibits or expresses the behaviour to a *high level*. There is clear (overt) evidence that the client is responding as intended to the therapist behaviours. The rater perceives that the client response is likely to have a substantial effect on client goal progress.

Table A.2 OPC-FM item descriptor and detailed rating guide

Fidelity item	Description	Rating guide
Critical components (items 1–9)		
1 **Therapist expresses empathy through comment & gesture, comprising non-judgmental responsiveness to the client's emotional experience.**	This item reflects the quality of therapist's use of empathy and is a key indicator of the quality of the therapeutic alliance. The rater considers verbal (e.g., utterances, tone of voice) and non-verbal (e.g., eye contact, nodding) gestures that indicate responsive, timely, and accurately pitched expression of empathy. Therapist's responses indicate non-judgemental acceptance of client's point of view and positive regard towards the client. The intended effect is that the client feels understood, with their experience acknowledged. However, the therapist is rated on their accurate *use* of empathy rather than the client's response (which is rated in item 12).	(0) Absent (1) Low • Therapist shows limited expression of emotion or interest in response to client (e.g., limited nodding, smiling, uttering). • May talk over client or make few responses when a response is warranted. • Low use of client's words – instead reframes experience or description in professional language. (2) Moderate • Therapist shows moderate expression of emotion, interest in response to client. • Some discernment by therapist between points of high meaning/emotionality to client but timing or magnitude of response may mismatch client need for empathy. • Authenticity of empathy may be unclear or mixed. (3) High • Therapist shows high level of genuine empathy for client including non-judgemental acceptance and attendance to their experiences. • Verbal and non-verbal responses are well timed and well pitched to match client need.

Table A.2 continued

Fidelity item	Description	Rating guide

2 **Therapist prompts client-led goal setting around a situation that is clearly highly meaningful to client.**	The therapist asks open-ended questions that invite the client to state their most valued current life goal. Invitations to goal statements are not prefaced with conditions (e.g., to fit a specific professional role). The therapist prompts goal clarification as often as is required for the client to articulate a goal that captures what is personally meaningful to them.
	
	The intended effect is that the goal reflects the client's current priority and core values. In doing so, the client's motivation for making changes toward goal achievement is high.
	
	Question examples include:
	
	• *What is most important for you right now?*
	• *What is your priority today?*
		(0) Absent
		(1) Low
		  • Therapist's questioning about goals is either too broad or too narrow to identify a clear but meaningful goal for the client.
		  • Therapist seems to 'miss the main point' that the client is trying to make.
		  • Therapist may attempt to shape goal statements into an area in which the therapist feels more comfortable.
		(2) Moderate
		  • Therapist asks questions that attempt to clarify the client's goal but misses important opportunities to ensure the goal is clear and highly meaningful to the client.
		  • Therapist may move into performance analysis questioning before goal is clearly stated.
		(3) High
		  • Therapist persists in questioning to clarify a meaningful goal until the goal is clear to both therapist and client.
		  • Therapist is able to use a wide range of questioning in order to clarify the goal when client becomes uncertain or vague.
		  • There is no attempt to influence the nature of the goal beyond that it is clear and meaningful.

Fidelity item	Description	Rating guide
3 **Therapist prompts occupation and participation-focused (activity + context) expression of the goal.**	The therapist prompts the client to describe how the goal is manifest in the activities and contexts of everyday life situations. The intended effect is to help the client to be very clear about what specifically they are seeking to be different in their occupational performance and participation. Question examples include: • *What will that look like?* • *How will you know when x is achieved?*	(0) Absent (1) Low • Therapist is unable to clarify the expression of the goal as an activity and in a specific context. • Therapist settles on goals that remain abstract, e.g., feeling better about something, describing a bodily function (e.g., 'stronger, co-ordinated') or skill-based (devoid of life context or situation). (2) Moderate • Therapist directs clarification of the activity and context expression of goals to some extent. Therapist may miss opportunities to clarify the goal activity and context. • Questions may lack specificity, thus having limited effect in clarifying the activity + context expression of the goal. • Questioning may move away from what is most meaningful to client in places. (3) High • Therapist asks specific questions to clarify the activity + context of goals while maintaining the meaningfulness of goals. • Therapist persists with goal clarification until the activity and context of goals is clear to both client and therapist.

Table A.2 continued

Fidelity item	Description	Rating guide
4 **The therapist prompts the client to envision the preferred, future goal situation.** **In subsequent sessions, the therapist refers to or prompts further clarification of the previously discussed vision.**	The therapist asks the client to describe and visualise goal achievement in considerable detail, including client's actions and interactions and the optimal environmental conditions. Although this item relates to therapist application of the envisioning technique rather than client's response (see item 13), the intended effect on client is that they visualise themselves enacting the achieved goal. In doing so it is intended that the client gains insight into how the goal could be achieved and mental rehearsal of the actions leading to goal achievement. Question examples include: • *Can you paint me a picture of what this will look like?* • *Imagine for a moment that there is no longer any problem and the goal is achieved. What do you notice is different?* • *Can you clarify x about how this will happen?*	(0) Absent (1) Low • The therapist uses only one question type (once, or repeatedly) to elicit client envisaging of the preferred future performance. • The therapist does not redirect the client if they digress into describing the problem situation or other topics not directly related to the goal. (2) Moderate • Therapist uses a narrow range of questions to optimise client's focus on the preferred future goal performance. • The tone of envisioning questioning may encourage a focus on facts rather than immersed visualisation (e.g., brisk, detached, lacking shared visualisation). • The therapist does some redirection of the client when they digress from describing the preferred future performance, but allows the client to spend considerable time describing problems, without attempting redirection. (3) High • Therapist uses a wide range of questions to optimise client's focus on the preferred future goal performance. • The tone of questioning encourages full immersed visualisation of the desired future performance. The therapist appears to also be visualising the desired future performance. • When the client perseverates on problem description, the therapist redirects the client to describing the preferred future performance or digresses to other topics with respect and patience.

Fidelity item	Description	Rating guide
5 **Performance analysis is oriented mostly to the preferred (goal) situation and solutions leading to it (i.e., performance analysis is not oriented to the problem or current situation).**	This item describes the therapist's orientation of discussion to the preferred goal situation rather than an orientation to the current (usually problem-oriented) situation. The orientation to the preferred (goal) situation is in contrast to a problem orientation in which a therapist might ask questions to fully understand the cause of the problem (e.g., a person's impairments or performance limitations). While this item is closely related to item 4 (envisioning) and item 6 (goal analysis), this item particularly captures the solution rather than problem orientation of therapist questioning. The intended effect on the client is to optimise their identification of strategies or changes towards goal achievement (since solutions tend to arise from describing the preferred future and not the current problem). Question examples include: • *I'm curious to hear more about what you think that would look like when you are back at work.* • *What would be happening instead, when the problem you've just described is not occurring?*	(0) Absent (1) Low • Questioning is mostly directed to describing the problem (current performance) rather than the goal (preferred performance). (2) Moderate • Questioning oscillates between directing the client to describe the problem (current performance) and the goal (preferred performance). (3) High • Questioning is almost exclusively directed to the client describing, reflecting on, or analysing the goal (preferred performance).

Table A.2 continued

Fidelity item	Description	Rating guide
6 **Therapist prompts client-led performance analysis of the goal situation. Prompts relate to client's perceptions and understanding of goal situations rather than therapist's understandings and perceptions.**	This item reflects therapist's use of questions and prompts that cue the client to lead a detailed analysis of goal achievement (referred to in OPC as collaborative performance analysis), considering how aspects of the person, task, and environment influence achievement of the goal situation. Distinct from item 4, the questions focus on *analysis* rather than *envisioning* of goal achievement. The intended effect on the client is active engagement in the analysis of development of insight into how goal progress can be made. Through this highly engaged learning process, the client is enabled to identify strategies with low levels of direct input from the therapist (see items 13 & 14). The client is also able to develop transferable skills in performance analysis related to their personal situation. Question examples include: • *When you say you think your child knows what to do, what makes you sure about this?* • *Could you talk me through how you would like to see this task happening at work? What are the steps?*	(0) Absent (1) Low • Questions relate to/extend the therapist's understanding rather than the client's insights. • Questions seem irrelevant or unrelated to the client. • The therapist provides an analysis of the situation (rather than asking questions) without seeking permission from the client. • The therapist may *overtly* attempt to persuade (i.e., hint at, influence, or persuade) the client into a particular analysis/interpretation of goal-related performance. (2) Moderate • The therapist asks a moderate range of questions to prompt the client's analysis of goal-related situations. Client reflection may be limited by an overly narrow range of questions. • Questions may be very abstract or worded using professional jargon that is difficult for the client to respond to. • The therapist may subtly attempt to persuade (i.e., hint at, influence, or persuade) the client into a particular analysis/interpretation of goal-related performance. • The therapist makes some attempt to follow the client's lead in the analysis but with some reluctance to drop their own line of enquiry.

Fidelity item	Description	Rating guide
		(3) High • The therapist asks a wide range of questions that prompt the client to consider how aspects of the person, task, and environment influence achievement of the goal situation. • Questions primarily relate to and extend client's understanding of the situation (rather than the therapist's). • The therapist is flexible in changing the line of enquiry in response to client's understanding and reflections, while maintaining a focus on analysis of the preferred future performance. • The therapist goes at the client's pace, accepting the level of reflection/insight that the client arrives at within the exchange (i.e., not rushing the client to a fuller conclusion or understanding) and modifying questioning to prompt further reflection and analysis as new insights are reached.

Table A.2 continued

Fidelity item	Description	Rating guide
7 **Therapist prompts client decision-making/choices about identifying and selecting solutions/strategies leading to goal achievement.**	This item describes the extent to which the therapist places agency with the client to make explicit choices in judgement or action that relate directly to goal progress. Distinct from item 6 (which focuses on client-led *analysis*, which may include descriptions, reflections, or musings), this item focuses on instances in which the client is prompted to *make a decision or choice.* The intended *effect on the client* is evident in items 13 & 14 when client's independence in analysis and decision-making on actions is evaluated. In contrast to the effect on the client, item 7 captures the *therapist's behaviour*, irrespective of how strongly the client responds to the behaviour. Question examples include: • *As you hear yourself describing these ideas, what seems most helpful to you at this point?* • *It sounds like you have a couple of choices here. What do your instincts tell you is most likely to work?*	(0) Absent (1) Low • The therapist offers very few opportunities to the client to make a decision or choice in the analysis of the goal situation or in deciding action to take. • The therapist may assume that the client agrees with them on either analysis or actions/strategies. • The therapist may be quite directive in what is discussed and/or what actions should be taken to progress goals. (2) Moderate • The therapist offers several opportunities for the client to make a choice in their opinion or action but also misses several opportunities. • The therapist may oscillate between cueing the client to make a choice/decision or being presumptuous or directive as to what opinion the client has or what action they will take. (3) High • The therapist consistently offers the client opportunities to state their judgement or choose a course of action. • The therapist is not directive or presumptive about the opinions, actions, or choices of the client.

Fidelity item	Description	Rating guide
8 **Therapist prompts client to specify details of their action plan (i.e., when, where, how, with whom).**	This item describes the therapist's use of questions that prompt the client to be very specific about their intended action. Distinct from item 7, which reflects the overall degree to which opportunities for choice were offered to the client, item 8 reflects questions that centre on specific action choices, once a general strategy has been decided on by the client. The intended effect is to optimise the likelihood that the client will enact the changes (including strategies) that they have stated. In contrast to the effect on the client, item 8 captures the *therapist behaviour*, irrespective of how strongly the client responds to the behaviour. These specific action questions are intended to uncover any as yet unstated potential barriers to action that need to be addressed or circumvented. Barriers may be external (such as the absence of needed equipment) or internal (such as negative self-talk). These questions also optimise the likelihood of action by refining client's visualisation of taking action. Question examples include: • *When do you think would be the best time to try out this idea? To give this your best shot, who would be important to have present, or to not be there?*	(0) Absent (1) Low • Therapist's questions related to client's enactment of strategies is vague and minimal. (2) Moderate • Therapist's questions related to client's enactment of strategies is somewhat specific and moderately thorough, but some steps of enactment (e.g., where, when, how, with whom) are unclear. • There may be some hesitancy from the client in acting on the plan that the therapist did not probe (but ideally would have). (3) High • Therapist's questions related to client's enactment of strategies is detailed and thorough with a very specific description from the client about where, when, how, and with whom they will enact the plan. • Any hesitancy indicated from the client at enacting the plan is probed and explored.

Table A.2 continued

Fidelity item	Description	Rating guide
9 **Therapist prompts client evaluation of planned strategies and outcomes after they are attempted. (Subsequent sessions only. Mark NA if first session.)**	This item describes therapist's questioning that explores client's evaluation of how well planned actions from a previous session were enacted or effective. The intended effect on the client is: • Positioning as the authority on what works to achieve their goal. • Remembering their intention to act. • Engaging in more detailed analysis and reflection based on their observations of what worked. • Acceptance and persistence when situations do not go as planned. Question examples include: • *How well do you think your strategy worked?* • *How well would you say your child is doing at playing alongside others now?*	NA (if first session) (0) Absent (1) Low • Therapist asks cursory or vague question as to how the plan worked. • Therapist assumes that the plan was implemented. • Therapist seems to have little interest in hearing that the plan may not have worked. • The therapist unilaterally states whether she thinks the plan worked. (2) Moderate • Therapist asks specific questions of the client's evaluation of how well a plan worked, however there may be lost opportunities to seek additional detail in what was enacted or how the client came to their conclusion of its effectiveness or otherwise. • The client is asked to judge whether the plan is working, but there may be some subtle coercion to reach a particular conclusion by the therapist. (3) High • The therapist asks specific questions of the client's evaluation of how well the planned worked. • The therapist responds openly, showing curiosity, about any difficulties implementing the plan and in client's evaluation of the plan (negative and positive). • The therapist asks follow-up questions as to how the client thinks the plan could be more fully enacted or altered (or if it should be abandoned). • The client is asked to judge whether the plan is working.

Fidelity item	Description	Rating guide
10 **Therapist prompts client generalising successful strategies to other valued activities, contexts, and roles.** **(Subsequent sessions only. Mark NA if first session.)**	This item reflects how thoroughly the therapist prompts the client to reflect on and enact generalisation of the strategy to other situations where it might be useful. This includes situations where other people might be encouraged to use the strategy, future situations, and other circumstances in which the strategy might need to be modified. The intended effect on the client is to prompt generalisation and transfer of successful strategies. Question examples include: • *Where else would this strategy be useful?* • *Who else that supports your wife could benefit from this strategy that seems to work well for you?*	NA (if first session) (0) Absent (1) Low • Therapist asks cursory or vague question as to how the strategy could be generalised. • The therapist assumes that the client will generalise the strategy. • The therapist tells the client how they could/should generalise the strategy. (2) Moderate • The therapist asks some questions as to how effective strategies could be generalised but does not persist to the extent that a specific response, likely to be enacted, is stated by the client. There is likely to be some effect on the client's future action but some opportunity to optimise this effect is lost. (3) High • The therapist asks specific and thorough questions as to how the client could apply the strategy in other situations including (but not exhaustively) alternative contexts, activities, roles, people, and into the future.

Table A.2 continued

Fidelity item	Description	Rating guide
Client response items (items 11–18)	*Note: Client level of response may not match the quality of the therapist's OPC behaviour. A therapist may execute an OPC behaviour very well yet it is not effective in eliciting a response due to client-specific conditions. Alternatively, a therapist may apply an OPC behaviour poorly or not at all yet the client spontaneously exhibits the intended behaviours described here. It is important to consider the degree of response separate to the quality of therapist's attempt to elicit each client response.*	
11 **The client seems to trust the therapist.**	This item describes the rater's impression of how relaxed, open, and trusting of the therapist the client appears. The client appears to feel respected, accepted without judgement. This is a particularly subjective judgement by the rater. Distinct from item 1, this item refers to the client's trust, rather than behaviours the therapist may have exhibited to engender trust. The intended effect is that the client is honest with therapist about their feelings and events related to goal achievement. This could be evident by: • The client appears relaxed with the therapist (unguarded). • The client talks openly with the therapist (high level of disclosure). • The client is comfortable to express emotion as it arises.	(0) Absent (1) Low • The client adopts distant or closed postures. • Their words are curt with no emotional expression. • The client sounds and appears guarded. (2) Moderate • The client appears fairly relaxed and partially guarded. • They may be open regarding information but with minimal emotional expression when difficult information is shared. (3) High • The client appears relaxed, open, expressive, and comfortable throughout the interaction, including during disclosure of difficult or emotive information.

Fidelity item	Description	Rating guide
12 **Client articulates specific reflection and analysis of goal-related situations.**	This item describes client's depth of reflection and analysis of goal-related situations. Distinct from other items, this item centres on reflection and analysis, rather than planning (item 13) and enacting (item 14). The intended effect on the client is heightening client's sense of competence and autonomy in understanding goal-related situations, thus increasing client's intrinsic motivation toward achieving their goals. Client-specific reflection and analysis could be evident as: Client: *When I think about it, I guess he [employer, child, partner] probably is a bit worried/uncertain/ frustrated. Really, he should know what is going to happen . . . [silence] . . . a big assumption, I guess.*	(0) Absent (1) Low • Client makes very vague/general statements about what they have observed of goal-related performance or their preferred future performance. • No new insight is evident. The client is unlikely to act differently in the coming week during goal-related activities. • No/limited silent periods during the session when the client appears to be thinking. (2) Moderate • There are silent periods during the session when the client appears to be thinking. • Client's comments indicate some reflection and insight but only to a moderate level. There may be some resistance/hesitancy to reflect more deeply. • There is likely to be some impact on client behaviour in the coming week that may impact goal progress but there is a sense that the reflection is unresolved. (3) High • There are silent periods during the session when the client is thinking. • Client's stated reflections and analysis are specific, clear, and evolving. • The client appears to answer their own question, or have an insight stimulated from their own reflection. • New learning in relation to goal situations is evident. • The client is very likely to act differently in the coming weeks, due to insights gained, in a way that is likely to impact goal progress.

Table A.2 continued

Fidelity item	Description	Rating guide
13 **Client articulates specific planned actions within goal-related activities outside of direct contact with therapist.**	This item reflects the clarity and specificity of the client's descriptions during sessions of what they intend to do differently to progress towards goal achievement. Clear and specific statements of intended actions are more likely to be implemented than vague statements. Distinct from item 14 (which addresses *enactment*), this item reflects *stated intended* actions. The intended effect on the client is greater commitment to enacting the plan, thus goal progress. This could be evident by: Client: *Tuesday night would be a good time to sit down with the family and plan this. We should turn off the T.V. – no devices.*	(0) Absent (1) Low • Client describes vague intended action; it is not entirely clear what will happen, where, how, or with whom. • It seems unlikely to the rater that the client will actually enact the plan. • The client's tone of voice indicates low enthusiasm for the plan, even though it is their idea. (2) Moderate • The client describes a somewhat specific plan. However it is not entirely clear what is intended to happen. • The client may not answer therapist's attempts to clarify the plan. • The client may appear conflicted (i.e., motivated but hesitant) as they describe the plan. (3) High • The client describes very clear and specific plans about when where, how, what, and with whom they will enact the plan. • It appears that the client is quite likely to attempt to enact the plan with conviction and perseverance.

Fidelity item	Description	Rating guide
14 **Client reports enacting actions intended to improve goal progress (including planned actions and innovations) in subsequent sessions. (Subsequent sessions only. Mark NA if first session.)**	This item describes client's exhibiting evidence of *enacting* plans or ideas discussed with the therapist. This may occur during the session (such as ways to support someone with physical disabilities to transfer from chair to toilet). Enacting of plans might also be illustrated by client's reporting of what was done between sessions, such as strategies to better manage the morning routine. Actions may have been an explicit part of the plan from prior session or may be new ideas that the client developed independently, but were intended to influence goal progress. This item is distinct from item 12 (which captures the extent that the client states what they *plan to do*). Item 14 instead captures what the client actually did. The intended effect on the client is goal progress and a developing sense of their own autonomy and competence in effecting change. Responses could include: Therapist: *So, what did you do differently since we last spoke?* Client: *I don't know really. I guess I just waited a bit longer before jumping in to help.* Therapist: *What happened as you tried to implement your plan from last week?* Client: *It was really hard. I was worried it would upset everyone. But I was determined to try. It did seem to help.*	NA (if first session) (0) Absent (1) Low • Client reports taking no or very limited action (planned or otherwise) intended to progress towards goal achievement. No effect on goal progress is anticipated based on client actions (observed or reported). (2) Moderate • Client reports taking some actions that were intended to progress towards goal achievement. • Action may have been with limited conviction or not sustained over the week, but some moderate effect on goal progress is anticipated from actions. (3) High • Client reports taking substantial and sustainable actions likely to significantly impact on goal progress.

Table A.2 continued

Fidelity item	Description	Rating guide
Distinguishing items (15–18)	*Note: The following items reflect what therapists attempting to implement OPC should not do. High scores in these items reflect low-quality implementation of OPC. A therapist may execute other OPC behaviours well and also engage in the following behaviours. This would reduce the therapist's overall fidelity score. Scores are reversed at the point of summating scores.*	

15 **Therapist provides advice without implicit or stated permission.**	This item describes therapist behaviours in which direct, unsolicited advice is provided by the therapist. Permission from the client is not sought by the therapist or stated.
	
	This item is the inverse of items 12 and 13.
	
	The effect on the client of direct unsolicited advice is likely to reduce their sense of their own competence and autonomy in self-managing goal-related situations.
	
	Examples include:
	
	• *What you need to do is . . .*
	• *Do you know about the x programme? It works really well in situations like this. Here, let me show you.*
		(0) Absent
		(1) Low [consistent with OPC]
		  • The therapist does not provide unsolicited advice.
		  • Any new information introduced by the therapist is preceded with the seeking of permission from the client to do so.
		  • Following information sharing, the client is asked to critique the information or decide if or how it could be applied to their circumstances.
		(2) Moderate
		  • Therapist provides advice with some attempt to obtain permission from the client, but does not wait for or clarify if permission is given. The therapist may either ask permission but then not check if the client found it valuable or plans to apply it.
		(3) High [inconsistent with OPC]
		  • Direct and unsolicited advice given.
		  • Therapist appears to assume (i.e., does not clarify) that the client wants the information and will apply it.

Fidelity item	Description	Rating guide
16 **Therapist attempts to persuade client to agree with therapist's interpretation or ideas.**	This item describes behaviours by the therapist that are intended to convince the client to agree with the therapist. They may be directed at any aspect of the discussion such as analysis of a situation, actions to take, or evaluation of the effects of any actions. Distinct from item 15 this item refers to the use of words or tone of voice to not just inform/advise (as in item 15) but to persuade or convince the client to agree with the therapist. The effect on the client may be either a distancing from the therapist (i.e., a loss of trust), lying to the therapist about their intention to act, or loss of client sense of autonomy and self-confidence. Examples include: Therapist: *I really think this is the best approach. You will give it a try, won't you? You see, [child] does prefer it like this, don't they?*	(0) Absent (1) Low [consistent with OPC] • No use of persuasion, covert (e.g., hinting) or overt (e.g., imploring, suggesting, or strongly recommending). • Therapist consistently allows client to retain their autonomy in making observations, evaluations, and choices. • Therapist may, with permission, offer information but does not attempt to influence client's opinion of the information. (2) Moderate • The therapist mostly allows the client to be the judge and make decisions throughout the session but with some subtle imposition of their authority in a way intended to sway client's stated opinions or actions. (3) High [inconsistent with OPC] • Therapist uses words and tone of voice to persuade or influence client at key points of analysis, decision-making, or evaluation. • Client sense of autonomy in making decisions is likely to be reduced as a result.

Table A.2 continued

Fidelity item	Description	Rating guide
17 **Therapist summarises or paraphrases the client's words in their own words, rather than using the client's words.**	This item describes therapist's use of their own wording to summarise, synthesise, or paraphrase what client has said or expressed. The effect on client may be a diminished sense of autonomy (i.e., control over the direction of the conversation) and competence in being able to articulate and understand situations fully. Examples include: Client: *I'm feeling lost, like things are hopeless.* Therapist: *You're in crisis. Your depression is really impacting on your ability to function.* Therapist: *So, there is some very different sensory processing going on here, and it is affecting multiple systems.*	(0) Absent (1) Low [consistent with OPC] • There may be some introduction of new words to extend client's reflection and insight, however this is brief. The client is invited to clarify or disagree with any brief summaries. • There is a sense that the client is the authority on their own lives. (2) Moderate • There is some use of client's words but this is augmented by therapist's language, paraphrasing client's expression in a way that directs authority to the therapist rather than the client. (3) High [inconsistent with OPC] • The therapist predominantly responds to the client using their own words to summarise the client's expression. • There is limited use of client's direct language. • There is a sense that the therapist is the expert, e.g., through lengthy description of client's circumstance or through use of professional language.

Fidelity item	Description	Rating guide

18 **Therapist uses 'hands-on' techniques (e.g., hand over hand) on the goal subject for the purposes of directly improving performance (excluding teaching or demonstrating a strategy to the client).**	This item describes the use of hands-on techniques by the therapist for the purposes of affecting change in goal-related performance. This excludes the use of techniques used with client's permission to demonstrate or explore the effectiveness of a technique that the client is interested in using.
	
	The effect on the client is likely to be a reduction in their sense of autonomy and competence in affecting goal achievement independently.
	
	Examples include:
	
	• Hand over hand
	• Movement facilitation
		(0) Absent
		(1) Low [consistent with OPC]
		  • Hands-on techniques are not used at all
		  • Hands-on techniques are used only with permission and for the purposes of collaborative exploration or teaching of client/others in the goal environment to use.
		  • No direct impact on goal progress is anticipated to have occurred from use of the hands-on techniques.
		(2) Moderate
		  • Hands-on techniques are used with permission, but outside of the purposes of collaborative exploration or teaching of client/others in the goal environment to use.
		(3) High [inconsistent with OPC]
		  • Hands-on techniques are used without permission or with the intention to directly impact goal progress.

Table A.3 OPC-FM summary score sheet

Rater ID:	Therapist:	Date scored:	Code:	Session #:
Goal: Who:	Activity:	Context:	Extent:	By when:

Summary self-reflection or feedback:

Critical Components	Quality rating					Items
	0	1	2	3	NA	
						1 Therapist expresses empathy through comment and gesture, comprising non-judgmental responsiveness to the client's emotional experience.
						2 Therapist prompts client-led goal setting around a situation that is clearly highly meaningful to client.
						3 Therapist prompts occupation and participation-focused (activity + context) expression of the goal.
						4 The therapist prompts the client to envision the preferred, future goal situation. In subsequent sessions, the therapist refers to or prompts further clarification of the previously discussed vision.
						5 Performance analysis is oriented mostly to the preferred (goal) situation and solutions leading to it. (i.e., performance analysis is not oriented to the problem or current situation).
						6 Therapist prompts client-led performance analysis of the goal situation. Therapist prompts relate to *client's perceptions* and understanding of goal situations rather than therapist's understandings and perceptions.

Rater ID:	Therapist:	Date scored:	Code:	Session #:
Goal: Who:	Activity:	Context:	Extent:	By when:

Summary self-reflection or feedback:

Items	Quality rating				
	0	**1**	**2**	**3**	**NA**
7 Therapist prompts *client decision-making*/choices about identifying and selecting solutions/strategies leading to goal achievement.					
8 Therapist prompts client to specify details of their action plan (i.e., when, where, how, with whom).					
Subsequent sessions only. Mark NA if first session.					
9 Therapist prompts *client evaluation* of planned strategies and outcomes after they are attempted.					
Subsequent sessions only. Mark NA if first session.					
10 Therapist prompts client generalising successful strategies to other valued activities, contexts, and roles.					
11 Client seems to trust the therapist.					
12 Client articulates specific *reflection and analysis* of goal-related situations.					
13 Client articulates specific *planned actions* within goal-related activities outside of direct contact with therapist.					
Subsequent sessions only. Mark NA if first session.					
14 Client reports *enacting actions* intended to improve goal progress (including planned actions and innovations) in subsequent sessions.					

Client Response

Table A.3 continued

Rater ID:	Therapist:	Date scored:	Code:	Session #:
Goal: Who:	Activity:	Context:	Extent:	By when:

Summary self-reflection or feedback:

	Quality rating				Items
	0	1	2	3	NA	
Distinguishing						15 Therapist provides advice without implicit or stated permission.
						16 Therapist attempts to persuade client to agree with therapist's interpretation or ideas.
						17 Therapist summarises or paraphrases the client's words in their own words, rather than using the client's words.
						18 Therapist uses 'hands-on' techniques (e.g., hand over hand) on the goal subject for the purposes of directly improving performance (excluding teaching or demonstrating a strategy to the client).
						COLUMN TOTALS

First session: (items 1–8; 11–13; 15–18)

Total score _____ /45 : _____ %

Subsequent session: (all items)

Total score _____ /54 : _____ %

Printable versions of this template are available at www.otago.ac.nz/opc.

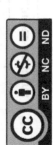

Appendix B: Occupational Performance Coaching process

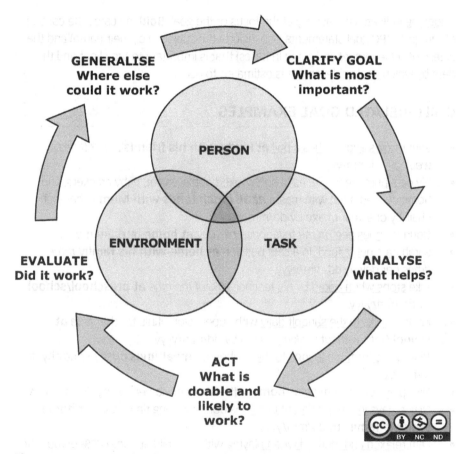

Figure B.1 Occupational Performance Coaching process

Source: First published Graham, F. (2020), Occupational Performance Coaching Resources. Retrieved from www.otago.ac.nz/opc (29/01/2020). This work is licensed under a Creative Commons Attribution-NonCommercial-NoDerivatives 4.0 International License. University of Otago. Reprinted with permission.

Appendix C: Occupational Performance Coaching: Goal examples

Underline indicates the activity at the focus of the goal. **Bold** indicates the context of the goal. OPC goal statements also include the subject (i.e., their name) and the *extent of achievement* (indicated in italics) that is important to the client and the date by which goal achievement is estimated to occur.

CHILD-RELATED GOAL EXAMPLES

- Sam <u>throws and catches a ball</u> **at kindy with his friends** *2 or 3 times a week* by dd/mm/yyyy.
- Ely <u>eats puree</u> (e.g., pieces of soft cooked apple, carrot, baby crackers, and home cooked meat with mash) ***at all lunch times*** **with Mum** in her high chair by one year of age by dd/mm/yyyy.
- Corinne <u>"goes pee"</u> *in the toilet once per day* **at home** by dd/mm/yyyy.
- Sarah <u>eats her 'x food'</u> in a safe position **at home with his family** *three times per day* by dd/mm/yyyy.
- Jake <u>stops when asked</u> by his teacher *90% of the time* **at preschool/school** by dd/mm/yyyy.
- Kahled <u>walks to the sandpit daily</u> with supervision of his teacher aide **at school** (*with/without walking frame*) by dd/mm/yyyy.
- Jane <u>walks from the lounge to the kitchen</u> for **mealtimes** *once per day* by dd/mm/yyyy.
- Nick <u>plays on his tummy</u> **at home with Mum** *twice per day* by dd/mm/yyyy.
- Oliver <u>plays in three different positions</u> during waking time, *daily*, **at home with his family** by dd/mm/yyyy.
- I am <u>relaxed and focused when playing</u> with my child at *home 80% of the time* (mother of a 12-month-old) by dd/mm/yyyy.
- My baby will be <u>settled and happy (not crying) during family routines</u> **at home** for *30 minutes per day* by dd/mm/yyyy. (Example of a mother's goal for a 12-month-old.)

ADULT-RELATED GOAL EXAMPLES

- Dave actively <u>participates in conversations</u> *50% of the time* during **social activities with friends** by dd/mm/yyyy.
- Sonya <u>walks **to the synagogue**</u> *"with confidence"* *once per week* for prayers by dd/mm/yyyy.
- Ethan <u>goes to a **baseball game**</u> **with friends** in Invercargill *(at least once)* by dd/mm/yyyy.
- Steve <u>does outdoor maintenance (raking and mowing lawn)</u> **at the cottage**, *at least once* by dd/mm/yyyy.
- Susan <u>organises collected pictures</u> of her life **on the computer** *to her own satisfaction* by dd/mm/yyyy.
- I <u>help my children with their homework</u> **after school, at home** *twice a week* by dd/mm/yyyy.
- I <u>mow my lawn</u> using ride-on lawn mower and *water potted plants* **at home** *once per week* by dd/mm/yyyy.
- I go <u>bushwalking with friends</u> in nearby **national park** *once per fortnight* by dd/mm/yyyy.
- I <u>participate in carpet bowls</u> weekly **at the seniors club** by dd/mm/yyyy.
- I <u>use my **mobile phone** to keep in touch</u> with my children and grandchildren *three times a week* by dd/mm/yyyy.
- I do my <u>weekly grocery shopping</u> **at the local supermarket** (home delivered) by dd/mm/yyyy.
- I <u>move sheep</u> from **pen to pen for shearing** *independently (excluding dog assistance)* during shearing season (dd/mm/yyyy).
- I <u>move cows</u> **between paddocks** using the farm truck (first gear only) *on a weekly basis* by dd/mm/yyyy.

Appendix D: Occupational Performance Coaching: Goal development example and template

Editable versions of this template are available at www.otago.ac.nz/opc.

Table D.1 Occupational Performance Coaching (OPC) goal development example

Goal component *Example*	Notes
Who? *Johnny*	Whose behaviour/ability are we seeking to change/improve? (This may be the client or their family, child, or dependent.) Client must have authority to try to effect this change (e.g., parent).
Will do what activity? *Will be seated on the mat*	What observable difference *will* occur (avoid stating what *won't* be done)?
In what daily life context? *During mat times at school*	Where will the change be observed? • Be specific. • Note that achieving change 'in clinic or during treatment session' is not the same as 'participating more fully in life'. The coachee must have authority in this context (e.g., teacher in classroom; parent at home).
How often/to what extent? *90% of the week (teacher report)*	How can the change be quantified? • Frequency • Level of satisfaction/experience • Length of time • Level of involvement • Intensity • Distance

Goal component *Example*	Notes
By when [DATE]? *the end of this term* *(dd/mm/yyyy)*	Agree to an estimated date that achievement of this goal is expected. This indicates when we expect to get a result, given the effort put in.
Complete goal statement: *Johnny will be seated on the mat during mat times at school 90% of the week (by teacher report) by the end of this term (dd/mm/yyyy).*	

Source: First published Graham, F. (2020), Occupational Performance Coaching Resources.

Retrieved from www.otago.ac.nz/opc (29/01/2020).

Table D.2 Occupational Performance Coaching (OPC) goal development template

Goal component	Notes
Who?	Whose behaviour/ability are we seeking to change/improve? (This may be the client or their family, child, or dependent.) Client must have authority to try to effect this change (e.g., parent).
Will do what activity?	What observable difference *will* occur (avoid stating what *won't* be done)?
In what daily life context?	Where will the change be observed? • Be specific. • Note that achieving change 'in clinic or during treatment session' is not the same as 'participating more fully in life'. The coachee must have authority in this context (e.g., teacher in classroom; parent at home).

Goal component	Notes
How often/to what extent?	How can the change be quantified? • Frequency • Level of satisfaction/experience • Length of time • Level of involvement • Intensity • Distance
By when [DATE]?	Agree to an estimated date that achievement of this goal is expected. This indicates when we expect to get a result, given the effort put in.
Complete goal statement:	

Source: First published Graham, F. (2020), Occupational Performance Coaching Resources.

Retrieved from www.otago.ac.nz/opc (29/01/2020).

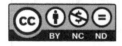

Appendix E: Suggested wording for Occupational Performance Coaching (OPC) Template for Intervention Description and Replication (TIDieR)

The Template for Intervention Description and Replication (TIDieR: (Hoffmann et al., 2014) provides suggested presentation of brief fidelity-related information in publications of OPC research. **The primary publication source for all items are (Graham, Rodger, & Ziviani, 2009) and (Graham, Kennedy-Behr, & Ziviani, 2020) with up-to-date information also provided at www.otago. ac.nz/opc**.

Table E.1 Suggested wording for Occupational Performance Coaching TIDieR

1 NAME **Occupational Performance Coaching (OPC)**
2 WHY OPC draws on dynamic systems perspectives of enablement, ecological perspectives of learning and behaviour change, and humanist and behaviour change principles to enhance client engagement in rehabilitation toward achieving personally valued occupational/participation goals.
3 WHAT MATERIALS The therapist uses no specialised equipment or materials. No standardised assessments or other assessment of impairments are used. No hands-on or directive (e.g., therapist arranging environment) methods are used with either the client or their dependent unless requested by the client in the context of context of trialling ideas within a coaching exchange.

4 WHAT PROCEDURES

OPC commences with questioning to identify clients' desired future state goals. Goals may not be directly related to health conditions or impairments. Goals are expressed at the level of observable action, comprising statement of an activity in a specific context which reflects personally meaningful change. Therapists consciously express empathy and listen mindfully to enhance the conditions for client trust in the therapist.

Therapists engage clients in a reflective discourse to explore potential actions that could lead to goal progress. Therapist questioning positions clients as knowledge holders and decision-makers, thus as agents of change. Therapists may provide specialist knowledge to clients only if clients give permission for this, if a knowledge gap is apparent after exploration of what clients already know. Goal progress is evaluated regularly with clients as the evaluator of change.

5 WHO PROVIDED

OPC can be applied by any rehabilitation professional with training in OPC. A minimum of 24 hours training is recommended for research using a mix of in-person and videoconference formats, enabling authentic clinical practice prior to completion of training.

6 HOW DELIVERED

OPC has been researched using in-person 1:1 or 1:family formats and through telephone/videoconference delivery.

7 WHERE

OPC is delivered in a private space such as client's home, workplace, or clinic setting.

8 WHEN and HOW MUCH

OPC can commence when clients have a concern or goal for themselves or their dependent.

OPC frequency is typically weekly or fortnightly but is at clients' discretion.

OPC sessions typically take 45–60 minutes but can range from 20 to 90 minutes.

Total number of sessions in research studies ranges from one to 12 sessions (average of five sessions). Sessions cease at goal achievement or a maximum of 12 sessions.

9 TAILORING

OPC questioning style is tailored to match client's language and cognitive ability and literacy level. For clients with significant cognitive impairment, OPC discourse is kept short and interspersed with active practice of goal-related activities.

10 MODIFICATIONS (During a study in response to study events)

NA as relates to study-specific events.

11 HOW WELL (Planned)

Quality of OPC delivery is assessed using the OPC Fidelity Measure (OPC-FM). Fidelity is assessed by therapists trained in OPC to an advanced level. Fidelity scores of >80% are estimated as required to elicit the desired client response.

12 HOW WELL (Actual)

Fidelity scores of delivered intervention should be reported with study findings.

Hoffmann, T. C., Glasziou, P. P., Boutron, I., Milne, R., Perera, R., Moher, D., . . . Johnston, M. (2014). Better reporting of interventions: Template for intervention description and replication (TIDieR) checklist and guide. *British Medical Journal, 348*, 1–12. doi:10.1136/bmj.g1687

Appendix F: Occupational Performance Coaching: Session Schedule

Editable versions of this template are available at www.otago.ac.nz/opc.

Table F.1 Session schedule for Occupational Performance Coaching (OPC)

Session Agenda	Question examples
SESSION 1: Goal, CPA[1], Action	
• **Establish valued participatory Goal**	• *What is most important to you right now?* • *What is your vision for you/your client/family?* • *If you were to change anything, what would it be?* • *What would have the biggest impact on you and your family/client?*
• **For highest priority goal, CPA collaboratively explores perceived bridges and barriers & client needs through to brief specific agreed Action plan.**	• *What happens now?* • *What have you tried already? How did that go?* • *What do you need to make this happen?* • *In relation to other things happening right now, how important is this to you?* • *What is your take-away plan from today's discussion?*

Session Agenda	Question examples
SESSIONS 2–12 (end at goal achievement): Goal, CPA, Action, Evaluate, Generalise	
• **Check Goal value each session**. • **Evaluate current performance compared to baseline from client perspective**. • **In light of Actions implemented and subsequent insights, continue CPA through to brief specific agreed Action plan**. • **Discuss opportunities to Generalise successful plans beyond immediate task, context, and people**. • **End when no further goals**.	• *Can I just check in with you, is this goal still your priority?* • *Given where you are at today, how important is achieving this goal to you right now?* • *What happened as you attempted . . . [specify plan]?* • *Tell me more about what happened as you tried to [implement strategy].* • *Where/when/who else might this strategy be relevant, or useful?*

Note: [1] CPA = collaborative performance analysis

Source: First published Graham, F. (2020), Occupational Performance Coaching Resources. Retrieved from www.otago.ac.nz/opc (29/01/2020). This work is licensed under a Creative Commons Attribution-NonCommercial-NoDerivatives 4.0 International License. University of Otago.

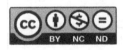

Appendix G: Occupational Performance Coaching: Casenote audit tool

Editable versions of this template are available at www.otago.ac.nz/opc.

Table G.1 Casenote audit tool

Audit date:		Therapist ID:	Client ID:	Session #:
Quality rating			**Item descriptor**	
NR	Unclear	Clear	Scoring notes: (0) if item is not reported; (1) if item is reported but meaning is unclear; (2) if item is clearly reported.	
0	1	2		
			1 The person who will engage in the goal activity is clearly stated (e.g., client, child, dependent).	
			2 Activity (task or routine) at the focus of the goal is stated.	
			3 Context of the goal is stated, e.g., home, school, work, specific community location.	
			4 Indication of the importance/value of the goal to the client. Revisited each session.	
			5 A specific score or descriptor related to client-valued gain in activity performance (e.g., quality/level of involvement, engagement, satisfaction). May be measured as frequency, duration, percent, or descriptively.	
			6 Specific date for anticipated goal achievement.	

| Audit date: | | Therapist ID: | Client ID: | Session #: |

Quality rating			Item descriptor
0	1	2	7 Brief description of current situation in relation to goal.
			8 Additional descriptors beyond goal statement of client vision. Highly valued and motivating aspects highlighted.
			9 Evidence of collaborative performance analysis: client-led observations, reflections, analysis related to achieving goal.
			10 In client words, statement of planned action in subsequent sessions.
			TOTAL SCORE if first session (Items 1–9): ___/18; = ___%
			11 Evidence that goal progress discussed. Specific reporting in relation to goal 'extent' documented at first session needed.
			12 Planned action specifically recorded. Success of strategies and/or rejection of earlier plans is noted.
			13 Evidence that opportunities to generalise successful plans noted.
			TOTAL SCORE if subsequent session (Items 1–13): ___/26; = ___%

Source: First published Graham, F. (2020), Occupational Performance Coaching Resources.

Retrieved from www.otago.ac.nz/opc (29/01/2020).

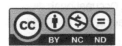

Appendix H: Occupational Performance Coaching: Casenote template

This appendix offers one exemplar of how casenotes for Occupational Performance Coaching may be reported and is not a required format for reports associated with OPC. Editable versions of this template are available at www.otago.ac.nz/opc.

Table H.1 Casenote template

DATE
GOAL *(who, what activity, where, how much, by when)*
CURRENT PERFORMANCE
PREFERRED PERFORMANCE
BRIDGES AND BARRIERS (*Person* *: Motivation, Knowledge;* **Task** *: Ability, Steps, Sequence, Standard;* **Environment** *: Social, Physical)*
ACTION PLAN *(who, do what?)*
NEXT MEETING

Source: First published Charles, L., Hamill, A., Graham, F. (2020), Occupational Performance Coaching Resources. Retrieved from www.otago.ac.nz/opc (29/01/2020).

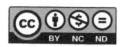

Appendix I: Occupational Performance Coaching: Discharge report template

This appendix offers one exemplar of how Occupational Performance Coaching may be reported and is not a required format for reports associated with OPC. Editable versions of this template are available at www.otago.ac.nz/opc.

REPORT

[Date]
[Client and other details required by service]

This report summarises [profession description] work undertaken between [date–date] with [client name] who was seen [number of sessions] times over [date period] in-person/via phone/via videoconference [delete as needed]. The primary intervention engaged in was Occupational Performance Coaching (OPC: Graham, Rodger, & Ziviani, 2009), which targets clients' personally valued goals in daily life activities and contexts. OPC prioritises client values, perceptions, and decisions on action in goal-related situations.

Graham, F., Rodger, S., & Ziviani, J. (2009). Coaching parents to enable children's participation: An approach for working with parents and their children. *Australian Occupational Therapy Journal, 56*(1), pp. 16–23.

[Client name] Goals

[Client name] identified the goals listed below in our work together. Goal progress was measured using the Canadian Occupational Performance Measure (COPM: Law et al., 2005), an interview-based self-assessment of success with performance of personally valued life activities and satisfaction with this performance. COPM scores are presented from our first and our last meeting, labelled 'before' and 'after' below. Change scores or two or more points are considered clinically significant (Law et al., 2005), however [client's name] description of change is a more sensitive indicator of change that occurred.

Law, M., Baptiste, S., Carswell, A., McColl, A., Polatajko, H., & Pollock, N. (2005). *COPM: Canadian Occupational Performance Measure* (4th ed.) Ottawa: CAOT Publications ACE.

Goal progress

Goal 1: [State the goal, including who, will do what activity, in what context, to what extent, by when]

[client's name] initially described [goal activity] performance as follows . . .

Through discussion and trialling of her/his ideas, [client's name] identified that the following adaptations/strategies/resources improved [who, doing what activity, in what context]. [Client's name] observed that [delete or expand as relevant] . . .

Over the past [length of time], [client's name] now reports that [who, can do what activity, in what context, to what extent]. [client's name] perceptions of goal success and satisfaction at the time of discharge from this service are reported above.

Goal 2: . . . [repeat as for goal 1 for all additional goals]

Table I.1 Client's evaluation of performance and satisfaction for each goal

#	Goal	COPM scores			
		Before		After	
		Perf*	Sat*	Perf	Sat
1	[who, will do what activity, in what context, to what extent, by when]				
2	[who, will do what activity, in what context, to what extent, by when]				
3	[who, will do what activity, in what context, to what extent, by when]				

Note Perf = client-rated evaluation of 'performance' of goal activity. Sat = client-rated evaluation of satisfaction with performance of goal activity.

Summary

Overall, [client's name] identified that key strategies for them that appeared to have wide applicability in their management of [x health-related situation] include [a, b, c].

While our work together has now concluded, [client's name] describes their future intentions in relation to these goals as [x, y, z].

We wish their every success in these endeavours.

[Sign here]

[Name, designation].

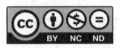

Index

Note: Page numbers in *italic* indicate a figure and page numbers in **bold** indicate a table or box on the corresponding page.